JCM-Advances in Cardiology

JCM-Advances in Cardiology

Editor

Michael Henein

MDPI • Basel • Beijing • Wuhan • Barcelona • Belgrade • Manchester • Tokyo • Cluj • Tianjin

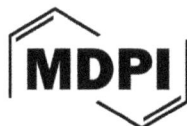

Editor
Michael Henein
Umeå University
Sweden

Editorial Office
MDPI
St. Alban-Anlage 66
4052 Basel, Switzerland

This is a reprint of articles from the Special Issue published online in the open access journal *Journal of Clinical Medicine* (ISSN 2077-0383) (available at: https://www.mdpi.com/journal/jcm/special_issues/JCM_Cardio).

For citation purposes, cite each article independently as indicated on the article page online and as indicated below:

LastName, A.A.; LastName, B.B.; LastName, C.C. Article Title. *Journal Name* **Year**, *Volume Number*, Page Range.

ISBN 978-3-0365-3345-2 (Hbk)
ISBN 978-3-0365-3346-9 (PDF)

© 2022 by the authors. Articles in this book are Open Access and distributed under the Creative Commons Attribution (CC BY) license, which allows users to download, copy and build upon published articles, as long as the author and publisher are properly credited, which ensures maximum dissemination and a wider impact of our publications.

The book as a whole is distributed by MDPI under the terms and conditions of the Creative Commons license CC BY-NC-ND.

Contents

About the Editor vii

Michael Y. Henein, Matteo Cameli, Maria Concetta Pastore and Giulia Elena Mandoli
COVID-19 Severity and Cardiovascular Disease: An Inseparable Link
Reprinted from: *J. Clin. Med.* **2022**, *11*, 479, doi:10.3390/jcm11030479 1

Sherif Ayad, Rafik Shenouda and Michael Henein
The Impact of COVID-19 on In-Hospital Outcomes of ST-Segment Elevation Myocardial Infarction Patients
Reprinted from: *J. Clin. Med.* **2021**, *10*, 278, doi:10.3390/jcm10020278 7

Michael Y. Henein, Ibadete Bytyçi, Rachel Nicoll, Rafik Shenouda, Sherif Ayad, Matteo Cameli and Federico Vancheri
Combined Cardiac Risk Factors Predict COVID-19 Related Mortality and the Need for Mechanical Ventilation in Coptic Clergy
Reprinted from: *J. Clin. Med.* **2021**, *10*, 2066, doi:10.3390/jcm10102066 15

Michael Y. Henein, Ibadete Bytyçi, Rachel Nicoll, Rafik Shenouda, Sherif Ayad, Federico Vancheri and Matteo Cameli
Obesity Strongly Predicts COVID-19-Related Major Clinical Adverse Events in Coptic Clergy
Reprinted from: *J. Clin. Med.* **2021**, *10*, 2752, doi:10.3390/jcm10132752 25

Filippos Triposkiadis, Andrew Xanthopoulos, Grigorios Giamouzis, Konstantinos Dean Boudoulas, Randall C. Starling, John Skoularigis, Harisios Boudoulas and Efstathios Iliodromitis
ACE2, the Counter-Regulatory Renin–Angiotensin System Axis and COVID-19 Severity
Reprinted from: *J. Clin. Med.* **2021**, *10*, 3885, doi:10.3390/jcm10173885 37

Giuseppe D'Angelo, David Zweiker, Nicolai Fierro, Alessandra Marzi, Gabriele Paglino, Simone Gulletta, Mario Matta, Francesco Melillo, Caterina Bisceglia, Luca Rosario Limite, Manuela Cireddu, Pasquale Vergara, Francesco Bosica, Giulio Falasconi, Luigi Pannone, Luigia Brugliera, Teresa Oloriz, Simone Sala, Andrea Radinovic, Francesca Baratto, Lorenzo Malatino, Giovanni Peretto, Kenzaburo Nakajima, Michael D. Spartalis, Antonio Frontera, Paolo Della Bella and Patrizio Mazzone
Check the Need–Prevalence and Outcome after Transvenous Cardiac Implantable Electric Device Extraction without Reimplantation
Reprinted from: *J. Clin. Med.* **2021**, *10*, 4043, doi:10.3390/jcm10184043 55

Valentina Ferradini, Joseph Cosma, Fabiana Romeo, Claudia De Masi, Michela Murdocca, Paola Spitalieri, Sara Mannucci, Giovanni Parlapiano, Francesca Di Lorenzo, Annamaria Martino, Francesco Fedele, Leonardo Calò, Giuseppe Novelli, Federica Sangiuolo and Ruggiero Mango
Clinical Features of LMNA-Related Cardiomyopathy in 18 Patients and Characterization of Two Novel Variants
Reprinted from: *J. Clin. Med.* **2021**, *10*, 5075, doi:10.3390/jcm10215075 65

Giovanni Peretto, Patrizio Mazzone, Gabriele Paglino, Alessandra Marzi, Georgios Tsitsinakis, Stefania Rizzo, Cristina Basso, Paolo Della Bella and Simone Sala
Continuous Electrical Monitoring in Patients with Arrhythmic Myocarditis: Insights from a Referral Center
Reprinted from: *J. Clin. Med.* **2021**, *10*, 5142, doi:10.3390jcm10215142 79

Abdulrahman Ismaiel, Mihail Spinu, Livia Budisan, Daniel-Corneliu Leucuta, Stefan-Lucian Popa, Bogdan Augustin Chis, Ioana Berindan-Neagoe, Dan Mircea Olinic and Dan L. Dumitrascu
Relationship between Adipokines and Cardiovascular Ultrasound Parameters in Metabolic-Dysfunction-Associated Fatty Liver Disease
Reprinted from: *J. Clin. Med.* **2021**, *10*, 5194, doi:10.3390/jcm10215194 . . . . **93**

About the Editor

Michael Henein is the Professor of Cardiology at Umeå University since 2010. He leads an International Cardiovascular Research program and has published over 400 papers in peer reviewed journals. He has written and edited many book chapters, including two chapters in the Oxford textbook of Medicine. He has graduated 20 PhD and 50 MSc students

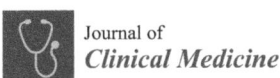

Editorial

COVID-19 Severity and Cardiovascular Disease: An Inseparable Link

Michael Y. Henein [1,2,*], Matteo Cameli [3], Maria Concetta Pastore [3] and Giulia Elena Mandoli [3]

1. Department of Public Health and Clinical Medicine, Umeå University, SE-901 87 Umea, Sweden
2. Molecular and Clinic Research Institute, St. George London & Brunel Universities, London SW17 0QT, UK
3. Department of Medical Biotechnologies, Division of Cardiology, University of Siena, 53100 Siena, Italy; matteo.cameli@yahoo.com (M.C.); pastore2411@gmail.com (M.C.P.); giulia_elena@hotmail.it (G.E.M.)
* Correspondence: michael.henein@umu.se

Citation: Henein, M.Y.; Cameli, M.; Pastore, M.C.; Mandoli, G.E. COVID-19 Severity and Cardiovascular Disease: An Inseparable Link. *J. Clin. Med.* **2022**, *11*, 479. https://doi.org/10.3390/jcm11030479

Received: 10 January 2022
Accepted: 13 January 2022
Published: 18 January 2022

Publisher's Note: MDPI stays neutral with regard to jurisdictional claims in published maps and institutional affiliations.

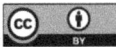

Copyright: © 2022 by the authors. Licensee MDPI, Basel, Switzerland. This article is an open access article distributed under the terms and conditions of the Creative Commons Attribution (CC BY) license (https://creativecommons.org/licenses/by/4.0/).

The COVID-19 pandemic is a global health issue that has so far affected over 250 million people worldwide. Having completed the first three waves of SARS-CoV2 infection, the world is currently facing the fourth wave, with significant consequences on overall global morbidity and mortality. The only effective proven weapons against COVID-19 are currently the vaccines and optimum prevention, in the form of personal protection, immune system strengthening with supplements, and personal isolation when tested positive. With this background, a thorough understanding of the viral mechanism of spread and underlying risk factors for critical disease is pivotal in order to limit COVID-19 detrimental consequences.

This Special Issue of the *Journal of Clinical Medicine* (JCM) entitled "Advances in Cardiology" offers four articles that contribute to the general physician and cardiologist's knowledge on the role of cardiovascular risk factors and angiotensin-converting enzyme-2 (ACE-2) in COVID-19 severity.

It is known that the presence of cardiovascular diseases (CVDs) is associated with worse clinical conditions and higher mortality in patients who contract COVID-19. Data analysis of 44,672 patients with COVID-19 found that a history of CVD provided a nearly fivefold increase in fatality rates when compared with patients without CVD (10.5 vs. 2.3%) [1]. Among approximately 9000 patients hospitalized for COVID-19 in North America, Europe, and Asia, 30.5% had hyperlipidemia, 26.3% had arterial hypertension, 14.3% had diabetes mellitus, 16.8% were former smokers, and 5.5% were current smokers. Additionally, 11.3% had coronary artery disease, and 2.1% had congestive heart failure [2]. A meta-analysis of 48,317 patients with COVID-19 confirmed that CVD and cardiovascular risk factors are closely associated with fatal outcomes, irrespective of age [3]. Other meta-analyses have also shown that the prevalence of arterial hypertension or cardiac disease was >15% and was associated with a higher need for critical care management. Hypertension has been shown to induce a pre-activation of the immune cells, with raised inflammatory cytokines, which led to a surging immune response in patients in contact with SARS-CoV2 and delayed viral clearance. Moreover, patients with diabetes mellitus and COVID-19 infection were at a higher risk of admission to the ICU and mortality due to hyperglycemia-associated vascular endothelial cell dysfunction [4]. Obesity has also been shown to have a key role in COVID-19 infection severity, because of its known associated inflammation that contributes to the weakening of the immune system by augmenting adipose tissue production of pro-inflammatory cytokines and downregulating anti-inflammatory immune cells.

Two of the studies published in this issue deal with a social category of people who are particularly at a high risk of exposure to SARS-CoV2 infection, i.e., clergy, because of the close inter-personal contact required during liturgies. Additionally, probably due to their special lifestyle, clergies are at significant risk because of the significantly high prevalence of

CV risk factors they carry, including hypertension, diabetes, and obesity. The two published studies are part of our multicenter "COVID-CVD study", which sought to investigate the importance of the various CV risk factors among Coptic clergies from Europe, the USA, and Egypt, in increasing their vulnerability to catching COVID-19, with its clinical consequences. In a group exceeding 1,600 clergies, the prevalence of SARS-CoV2 infection was 16.2%. Additionally, a model combining CV risk factors (hypertension, i.e., systolic blood pressure (SBP) $\geq$160 mmHg, diabetes mellitus, obesity, and history of coronary heart disease) was the most powerful independent predictor of COVID-19-related mortality, OR 3.991 ((1.919 to 6.844); p = 0.002) and the need for mechanical ventilation (OR 1.501 ((0.809 to 6.108); p = 0.001) [5]. In the second analysis, we found that obesity was the highest prevalent CV risk factor among Coptic clergies (above all, among Egyptians) and was the most powerful independent predictor of major COVID-19-related adverse events in the form of death or mechanical ventilation (OR = 4.180; 2.479 to 12.15; p = 0.01) [6]. These findings highlight the need for special attention to be given to clergy as a social category example for optimum protection from COVID-19 complications, with a serious need for lifestyle optimization and immune system support. Additionally, a well-designed education program for clergies is highly recommended, in order to optimally adhere to SARS-CoV2 contagion preventive measures and optimum control of CV risk factors according to available guidelines.

The Position Paper from VAS-European Independent Foundation in Angiology/Vascular Medicine for the Management of Patients with Vascular Disease or CV risk factors and COVID-19 suggested that lock-down policies for epidemic waves should target, in particular, patients with underlying CVD who should also undergo regular medical follow-up. They also recommended encouraging the use of telemedicine whenever possible, to improve adherence to antihypertensive, lipid-lowering, and hypoglycemic treatment according to current guidelines. It also recommends patients with underlying CVD and non-severe COVID-19 receive medical care at home, close follow-ups, and be prioritized for hospital admission when needed.

With respect to anti-hypertensive treatment, the role of ACE-inhibitors has been extensively sought during the pandemic, since the aminopeptidase angiotensin-converting enzyme 2 (ACE2) has been identified as a receptor for SARS-CoV2, due to its binding to the spike protein of the virus. The review by Triposkiadis et al. [7], included in this issue, elucidates the role of ACE2 in COVID-19 progression and severity, reassuring the scientific community on the safety of continuing the use of ACE inhibitors.

In fact, ACE2 is highly expressed in many organs such as cardiomyocytes, enterocytes, renal tubular cells, and sinonasal cavity cells, whereas in the lungs, the ACE2 expression is minimum. However, the expression of ACE2 depends on the immune responses; therefore, binding of ACE2 with SARS-CoV2 may amplify inflammatory signaling and ACE2 expression, as well as promote virus replication, its entrance into the host cell, and its spread throughout the organism with the contribution of inflammatory M1 macrophages, which, in turn, have marked upregulation of ACE2 on their surface. Therefore, each action promoting the expression of ACE2 instead of its inhibition may be harmful to COVID-19 progression in the organism after SARS-CoV2 infection. The authors of this article also illustrate, in detail, the peculiar impact of COVID-19 and the role of the renin–angiotensin–aldosterone system in specific populations, such as patients with cancer, renal failure, and chronic obstructive pulmonary disease. Mechanism and disease-specific risk factors are described, such as tumor stage, disease progression, and type of cancer (above all thoracic), which are high-risk factors for disease severity in cancer patients. Again, the role of CV risk factors is highlighted with obesity and diabetes mellitus, resulting in an imbalance in the renin–angiotensin–aldosterone system, with higher ACE2 expression, which leads to slower viral clearance. In the end, emerging therapies targeting transmembrane protease, serine 2 (TMPRSS2), and ACE2 co-factor involved in the SARS-CoV2 binding and internalization are introduced, which represent new therapeutic frontiers against COVID-19.

The fourth article addresses an important in-hospital issue, which is the outcome of ST-elevation myocardial infarction, hence impacting the national health services and national health systems. Our hospital admission analysis showed a trend toward a reduction in acute coronary syndromes incidence, with a substantial increase in STEMI fatality rate and complications during the pandemic, compared with 2019 [8]. This was explained by the decrease in percutaneous coronary intervention (PCI) procedures [9], with an annual 634 PCI patients falling by 25.7% during the COVID-19 period (mean 30.0 ± 4.01 vs. 40.4 ± 5.3 case/month) and prolongation of the time from first medical contact to needle (125.0 ± 53.6 vs. 52.6 ± 22.8 min, $p = 0.001$). Such significant change in practice was interpreted on the basis of patients' fear of visiting the hospital, lack of organized emergency pathways for acute coronary syndromes during the COVID-19 period, and occasional misdiagnosis in patients with respiratory symptoms. The last finding was higher in-hospital mortality (7.4 vs. 4.6%, $p = 0.036$), incidence of reinfarction (12.2 vs. 7.7%, $p = 0.041$), and the need for revascularization (15.9 vs. 10.7%, $p = 0.046$) during the COVID-19 pandemic. In fact, a dramatic increase in hospitalization for subacute myocardial infarction >72 h has been described worldwide, with increasing incidence of malignant arrhythmias and severe heart failure resistant to conventional therapy and often requiring inotropic or mechanical support. Untreated myocardial infarction is known to increase left ventricular maladaptive remodeling and the long-term incidence of dilated cardiomyopathy and heart failure. This would unavoidably constitute a clinical challenge and result in a poor prognosis. Possible solutions rely on optimal organization of healthcare services during the pandemic, social education, and alternative methods of follow-up to balance between the prevention of COVID-19 and acute coronary syndromes, such as the aforementioned telemedicine.

Beyond coronary heart disease, since many cases were described as due to SARS-CoV2 infection or vaccine induced (the former with a 40-fold higher incidence than the latter), which may also be a potential confounder of an acute coronary syndrome—namely, acute myocarditis. In severe cases, these may cause life-threatening ventricular arrhythmias; therefore, arrhythmia monitoring may be crucial for these patients. Peretto G. et al. [10] conducted a study in 104 adult patients with biopsy-proven active myocarditis and de novo ventricular arrhythmias, who underwent prospective monitoring by both sequential 24 h Holter ECGs and continuous arrhythmia monitoring (CAM), including either implantable cardioverter defibrillator (ICD) (60%) or loop recorder (40%). The authors found that nearly half of the patients developed ventricular arrhythmias over long-term follow-up, CAM was more accurate in the identification of patients with ventricular arrhythmias, and histological signs of chronically active myocarditis (70%) and anteroseptal late gadolinium enhancement (25%) were significantly associated with the occurrence of ventricular tachycardia. These important findings may help the decision-making processes in patients presenting with acute myocarditis.

Another consequence of myocarditis is the development of dilated cardiomyopathy (DCM), a complex disease for its variable etiology, complications, and management, irrespective of the etiology of DCM, primary, congenital/hereditary, or secondary, often a consequent to ischemic heart disease, myocarditis, infective or peripartum cardiomyopathy. Primary or secondary DCM may be complicated by valvular heart disease, chronic heart failure, arrhythmias, leading to sudden cardiac death; however, there are some primary forms that are particularly prone to develop arrhythmias, often presenting with sudden cardiac death, such as those deriving from LMNA gene (encoding for laminin A/C) mutation. The article by Ferradini et al. included in this issue [11] describes, among 77 families with DCM referred for genetic counseling and molecular screening, how they found 18 patients with heterozygotes mutation for laminin A/C with 2 new variants of the gene. Interestingly, 44.5% of patients presented with ventricular arrhythmias as the first symptom. These results highlight the importance of genetic analysis when laminin A/C mutation may be suspected in order to provide a good risk stratification of sudden cardiac death. In fact, there is currently a lack of targeted therapy for the treatment of LMNA variants-associated cardiomyopathy and the only therapy to consider is the prevention with ICD, also in these cases, because of the high risk of SCD in these patients.

It should be highlighted that ICD implantation is not free of risks. It carries a risk of pocket infection and leads to endocarditis with possible systemic infection, pneumothorax, or bleeding. It may also require new intervention either years after the first implantation, for example, to replace the battery, or earlier in the case of lead dislodging or for infections/malfunctions. While battery replacement without lead extraction is an almost simple procedure with only a few potential complications, transvenous lead extraction (TVE) is a challenging procedure that carries a high risk of life-threatening complications, such as superior vena cava tear, pericardial effusion, tamponade, and embolization. Therefore, a reconsideration of ICD indications is often operated when TVE should be performed, as recommended by the guidelines [12]. In this issue, D'Angelo et al. reported a study on 223 patients undergoing TVE, in 14.8% of whom no reimplantation was performed. At a median follow-up of 41 months, 11.8% received a new ICD after 17–84 months due to arrhythmic events. While hospitalization for device revision (in the reimplantation group) or late reimplantation (in the no-reimplantation group) was similar (11.1% vs. 12.1%, $p = 0.771$), as was short-term survival, five-year survival was significantly lower in the no-reimplantation group (78.3% vs. 94.7%, $p = 0.014$), and death occurred mostly for non-cardiac causes [13]. The absence of atrioventricular blocks in the primary indication and higher left-ventricular ejection fraction represented independent predictors favoring no-reimplantation. Therefore, these two elements may help therapeutic decisions, as these results recommend careful consideration of ICD reimplantation when TVE should be performed.

Finally, the eighth article in this Special Issue of Advances in Cardiology concerns a new but still important and timely topic, since the traditionally known non-alcoholic fatty liver disease, currently called metabolic-dysfunction fatty live disease (MAFLD), remains a challenging hepatic syndrome. Although its association with CV risk factors is well known, the mechanisms of its direct/indirect link with the CV system are still to be ascertained. In their article, Ismaiel et al. [14] investigated the association between adipokines, peptides product of the adipose tissue, and CV ultrasound parameters in 80 patients with hepatic steatosis evaluate by both hepatic ultrasonography and SteatoTestTM (40 patients with MAFLD diagnosis, 40 controls), who all underwent echocardiography and carotid Doppler ultrasound and adipokines analysis. The authors found that adiponectin and visfatin levels were not significantly different in MAFLD vs. controls. Visfatin was associated with mean carotid intima-media thickness, while adiponectin was associated with left ventricular ejection fraction and early/late diastolic waves (E/A) ratio in controls. A significant direct proportional association was found between adiponectin and E/A ratio in the univariate linear regression analysis but was lost in multivariate models. Conversely, although left ventricular ejection fraction was not significantly associated with adiponectin in univariate analysis, a significant inversely proportional association was demonstrated after adjustment using multivariate regression models, according to similar previous studies. These results may generate interesting hypotheses on the relationship between MAFLD and the CV system, but this needs to be further tested.

In conclusion, the articles in this issue are expected to assist the readers confronted by COVID-19 patients and guide them to pay particular attention to CV risk factors and lifestyle. They also highlight the relationship between the COVID-19 pandemic and other cardiac syndromes, as well as its potential cardiovascular clinical consequences and their predictors, which, in some cases, could be avoided.

Funding: This research received no external funding.

Conflicts of Interest: The authors declare no conflict of interest.

References

1. Wu, Z.; McGoogan, J.M. Characteristics of and important lessons from the coronavirus disease 2019 (COVID-19) outbreak in China: Summary of a report of 72314 cases from the Chinese Center for Disease Control and Prevention. *JAMA* **2020**, *323*, 1239–1242. [CrossRef] [PubMed]
2. Fried, J.A.; Ramasubbu, K.; Bhatt, R.; Topkara, V.K.; Clerkin, K.J.; Horn, E.; Rabbani, L.; Brodie, D.; Jain, S.S.; Kirtane, A.J.; et al. The variety of cardiovascular presentations of COVID-19. *Circulation* **2020**, *141*, 1930–1936. [CrossRef] [PubMed]
3. Bae, S.; Kim, S.R.; Kim, M.N.; Shim, W.J.; Park, S.M. Impact of cardiovascular disease and risk factors on fatal outcomes in patients with COVID-19 according to age: A systematic review and meta-analysis. *Heart* **2021**, *107*, 373–380. [CrossRef] [PubMed]
4. Al-Kuraishy, H.M.; Al-Gareeb, A.I.; Alblihed, M.; Guerreiro, S.G.; Cruz-Martins, N.; Batiha, G.E. COVID-19 in Relation to Hyperglycemia and Diabetes Mellitus. *Front. Cardiovasc. Med.* **2021**, *8*, 644095. [CrossRef] [PubMed]
5. Henein, M.Y.; Bytyçi, I.; Nicoll, R.; Shenouda, R.; Ayad, S.; Cameli, M.; Vancheri, F. Combined Cardiac Risk Factors Predict COVID-19 Related Mortality and the Need for Mechanical Ventilation in Coptic Clergy. *J. Clin. Med.* **2021**, *10*, 2066. [CrossRef] [PubMed]
6. Henein, M.Y.; Bytyçi, I.; Nicoll, R.; Shenouda, R.; Ayad, S.; Vancheri, F.; Cameli, M. Obesity Strongly Predicts COVID-19-Related Major Clinical Adverse Events in Coptic Clergy. *J. Clin. Med.* **2021**, *10*, 2752. [CrossRef] [PubMed]
7. Triposkiadis, F.; Xanthopoulos, A.; Giamouzis, G.; Boudoulas, K.D.; Starling, R.C.; Skoularigis, J.; Boudoulas, H.; Iliodromitis, E. ACE2, the Counter-Regulatory Renin–Angiotensin System Axis and COVID-19 Severity. *J. Clin. Med.* **2021**, *10*, 3885. [CrossRef] [PubMed]
8. Cameli, M.; Pastore, M.C.; Mandoli, G.E.; D'Ascenzi, F.; Focardi, M.; Biagioni, G.; Cameli, P.; Patti, G.; Franchi, F.; Mondillo, S.; et al. COVID-19 and Acute Coronary Syndromes: Current Data and Future Implications. *Front. Cardiovasc. Med.* **2021**, *7*, 593496. [CrossRef] [PubMed]
9. Ayad, S.; Shenouda, R.; Henein, M. The Impact of COVID-19 on In-Hospital Outcomes of ST-Segment Elevation Myocardial Infarction Patients. *J. Clin. Med.* **2021**, *10*, 278. [CrossRef] [PubMed]
10. Peretto, G.; Mazzone, P.; Paglino, G.; Marzi, A.; Tsitsinakis, G.; Rizzo, S.; Basso, C.; Della Bella, P.; Sala, S. Continuous Electrical Monitoring in Patients with Arrhythmic Myocarditis: Insights from a Referral Center. *J. Clin. Med.* **2021**, *10*, 5142. [CrossRef] [PubMed]
11. Ferradini, V.; Cosma, J.; Romeo, F.; De Masi, C.; Murdocca, M.; Spitalieri, P.; Mannucci, S.; Parlapiano, G.; Di Lorenzo, F.; Martino, A.; et al. Clinical Features of LMNA-Related Cardiomyopathy in 18 Patients and Characterization of Two Novel Variants. *J. Clin. Med.* **2021**, *10*, 5075. [CrossRef] [PubMed]
12. Kusumoto, F.M.; Schoenfeld, M.H.; Wilkoff, B.L.; Berul, C.I.; Birgersdotter-Green, U.M.; Carrillo, R.; Cha, Y.M.; Clancy, J.; Deharo, J.C.; Ellenbogen, K.A.; et al. 2017 HRS expert consensus statement on cardiovascular implantable electronic device lead management and extraction. *Heart Rhythm.* **2017**, *14*, e503–e551. [CrossRef] [PubMed]
13. D'Angelo, G.; Zweiker, D.; Fierro, N.; Marzi, A.; Paglino, G.; Gulletta, S.; Matta, M.; Melillo, F.; Bisceglia, C.; Limite, L.R.; et al. Check the Need–Prevalence and Outcome after Transvenous Cardiac Implantable Electric Device Extraction without Reimplantation. *J. Clin. Med.* **2021**, *10*, 4043. [CrossRef] [PubMed]
14. Ismaiel, A.; Spinu, M.; Budisan, L.; Leucuta, D.-C.; Popa, S.-L.; Chis, B.A.; Berindan-Neagoe, I.; Olinic, D.M.; Dumitrascu, D.L. Relationship between Adipokines and Cardiovascular Ultrasound Parameters in Metabolic-Dysfunction-Associated Fatty Liver Disease. *J. Clin. Med.* **2021**, *10*, 5194. [CrossRef] [PubMed]

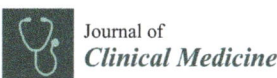

Article

The Impact of COVID-19 on In-Hospital Outcomes of ST-Segment Elevation Myocardial Infarction Patients

Sherif Ayad [1,*], Rafik Shenouda [2] and Michael Henein [3]

1 Faculty of Medicine, Alexandria University, Alexandria 21526, Egypt
2 International Cardiac Center, Alexandria 21526, Egypt; rafikbotros17@hotmail.com
3 Institute of Public Health and Clinical Medicine, Umea University, SE-90187 Umea, Sweden; michael.henein@umu.se
* Correspondence: sherifwagdyayad@yahoo.com; Tel.: +20-12-2226-4878

Abstract: Primary percutaneous coronary intervention (PPCI) is one of the important clinical procedures that have been affected by the COVID-19 pandemic. In this study, we aimed to assess the incidence and impact of COVID-19 on in-hospital clinical outcome of ST elevation myocardial infarction (STEMI) patients managed with PPCI. This observational retrospective study was conducted on consecutive STEMI patients who presented to the International Cardiac Center (ICC) hospital, Alexandria, Egypt between 1 February and 31 October 2020. A group of STEMI patients presented during the same period in 2019 was also assessed (control group) and data was used for comparison. The inclusion criteria were established diagnosis of STEMI requiring PPCI. A total of 634 patients were included in the study. During the COVID-19 period, the number of PPCI procedures was reduced by 25.7% compared with previous year (mean 30.0 ± 4.01 vs. 40.4 ± 5.3 case/month) and the time from first medical contact to Needle (FMC-to-N) was longer (125.0 ± 53.6 vs. 52.6 ± 22.8 min, $p = 0.001$). Also, during COVID-19, the in-hospital mortality was higher (7.4 vs. 4.6%, $p = 0.036$) as was the incidence of re-infarction (12.2 vs. 7.7%, $p = 0.041$) and the need for revascularization (15.9 vs. 10.7%, $p = 0.046$). The incidence of heart failure, stroke, and bleeding was not different between groups, but hospital stay was longer during COVID-19 (6.85 ± 4.22 vs. 3.5 ± 2.3 day, $p = 0.0025$). Conclusion: At the ICC, COVID-19 pandemic contributed significantly to the PPCI management of STEMI patients with decreased number and delayed procedures. COVID-19 was also associated with higher in-hospital mortality, rate of re-infarction, need for revascularization, and longer hospital stay.

Keywords: ST segment elevation myocardial infarction; COVID-19; primary percutaneous intervention

Citation: Ayad, S.; Shenouda, R.; Henein, M. The Impact of COVID-19 on In-Hospital Outcomes of ST-Segment Elevation Myocardial Infarction Patients. *J. Clin. Med.* **2021**, *10*, 278. https://doi.org/10.3390/jcm10020278

Received: 1 December 2020
Accepted: 11 January 2021
Published: 14 January 2021

Publisher's Note: MDPI stays neutral with regard to jurisdictional claims in published maps and institutional affiliations.

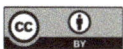

Copyright: © 2021 by the authors. Licensee MDPI, Basel, Switzerland. This article is an open access article distributed under the terms and conditions of the Creative Commons Attribution (CC BY) license (https://creativecommons.org/licenses/by/4.0/).

1. Introduction

Currently, primary percutaneous coronary intervention (PPCI) is the best management strategy for patients presenting with ST-segment elevation myocardial infarction (STEMI) according to the latest guidelines [1]. Studies have shown that time delay in PPCI has negative impact on the clinical outcomes of STEMI patients [2,3].

COVID-19 affected many aspects of human life since its start in early 2020, one of which is prioritizing clinical management of various medical conditions including coronary artery disease, particularly acute coronary syndrome and urgent interventions required for STEMI, a potential life-threatening condition. The WHO classifies COVID-19 cases into four categories based on clinical history, presentation, and laboratory findings: confirmed (COVID-19 +), suspected (COVID-19 +/−), contact (COVID-19 C), or non-suspected (COVID-19 NS) [4].

COVID-19 has significantly impacted conventional management of STEMI patients, resulting in practice variabilities between countries. Some countries have changed their reperfusion strategy to fibrinolytic therapy [5–7], others still follow the guidelines in performing PPCI to all STEMI patients [8–11]. The delay in seeking medical advice during the lockdown periods, the time needed for screening for COVID-19 infection, and the fear of healthcare providers regarding cross-infection are the main causes behind the change of practice of managing STEMI patients and the fall in PPCI procedures according to some reports [12–15].

In this study, we aimed to assess the impact of COVID-19 on in-hospital clinical outcome of STEMI patients managed with PPCI.

2. Experimental Section

2.1. Study Design

This is a retrospective observational study conducted on consecutive STEMI patients who presented to the International Cardiac Center (ICC) hospital, Alexandria, Egypt between 1 February and 31 October 2020. The inclusion criteria were established diagnosis STEMI (ST segment elevation more than 1 mm in two consecutive leads or new left bundle branch block associated with typical chest pain with or without elevated cardiac markers) fulfilling guidelines recommendation for PPCI treatment [1,16]. The exclusion criteria were previous CABG, cardiogenic shock, previous PCI of the same culprit vessel and severe left main (LM) coronary artery disease. Data from a group of STEMI patients who presented to ICC during the same period of 2019 was used for comparison, as control. Twenty patients in group A and 5 patients in group B were excluded. The study population included 634 patients who were classified into two groups:

Group A: Included 364 STEMI patients treated with PPCI before COVID-19 (year 2019).
Group B: Included 270STEMI patients treated with PPCI during COVID-19 (year 2020).

2.2. Data Collection

All patients' demographic data were collected including age, gender, comorbidities (hypertension, diabetes, dyslipidemia), obtained PPCI procedure details including time from symptom onset to first medical contact (FMC), and time from first medical contact to needle (FMC-to-N). From coronary angiograms the following information were collected; the culprit artery, number of diseased vessels, the use of antithrombotic treatment (acetyl salicylic acid, clopidogrel, ticagrelor, heparin, enoxaparin, and glycoprotein IIb/IIIa inhibitors), balloon pre-dilatation, stent details (number, length, and diameter), Thrombolysis In Myocardial Infarction (TIMI) score, flow at the end of the procedure, and duration of hospital stays. Also, any subsequent procedure related complications—e.g., heart failure, stroke, or bleeding—were documented.

2.3. Endpoint Measurements

The primary clinical outcomes were the percentage of PPCI procedures performed before and during the COVID-19 and the median time of first medical contact to needle (FMC-to-N), while the secondary outcomes were in-hospital mortality, major adverse cardiac and cerebrovascular events (MACCE) during hospital stay and the duration of hospitalization. MACCE was defined as death, re-infarction, need for revascularization, heart failure, stroke, and bleeding.

2.4. Statistical Analysis

Statistical Package for Social Sciences (SPSS version 20.0. IBM Corp, Armonk, NY, USA) was used for data analysis [17]. We described qualitative data using numbers and percentage. For quantitative data we used range (minimum and maximum), mean, standard deviation, and median. Chi-square test was used to compare categorical variables between different groups. Fisher's exact probability or Monte Carlo correction for Chi-square were used when more than 20% of the cells have expected count less than 5. Mann-Whitney test was used to compare groups for abnormally distributed quantitative variables. A p-value of <0.05 was considered significant for all tests.

An informed consent was obtained from every patient or the legal guardians. The study was approved by the local ethics committee (approval number 0304893).

3. Results

3.1. Patients Characteristics and Number of Procedures

During the COVID-19 period, the number of PPCI procedures was reduced by 25.7% compared with previous year (30.0 ± 4.01 vs. 40.4 ± 5.3 case/month). Both patient groups (A and B) were well matched with respect to demographic data and clinical characteristics with no significant difference between them. Only eight patients in group A and five patients in group B were more than 65–70 years of age. The baseline characteristics of both groups are presented in Table 1.

Table 1. Baseline characteristics, laboratory findings, procedural characteristics of the studied populations.

	Group A n = 364		Group B n = 270		p-Value
Age					
Range	36–88		35–82		0.568
Mean ± S.D.	58.9 ± 13.35		57.1 ± 12.60		
Gender					
Male	312	85.7%	220	81.5%	0.607
Female	52	14.3%	50	18.5%	
Risk factors					
Diabetes mellitus	130	35.7%	95	35.2%	0.521
Hypertension	156	42.9%	107	39.6%	0.411
Dyslipidemia	182	50.0%	122	45.2%	0.501
Smoking	208	57.1%	123	45.6%	0.364
Troponin					
Range	0.003–8.68		0.01–10.0		0.078
Mean ± S.D.	1.07 ± 2.21		1.65 ± 2.62		
CKmb					
Range	1.27–261.9		1.32–270.0		0.105
Mean ± S.D.	115.94 ± 76.29		124.3 ± 58.9		
Haemoglobin					
Range	9.3–17.1		9.5–16.0		0.524
Mean ± S.D.	13.87 ± 1.85		13.9 ± 1.71		
Lymphocytes					
Range	12–36		8–25		0.012 *
Mean ± S.D.	18.6 ± 6.21		14.78 ± 5.85		
D dimer					
Range	130–500		152–1500		0.0031 *
Mean ± S.D.	302.0 ± 132.17		505.6 ± 201.3		
Serum ferritin					
Range	72.0–135.0		85.0–166.0		0.011 *
Mean ± S.D.	93.48 ± 39.8		118.5 ± 42.51		
Serum creatinine					
Range	0.59–4.03		0.60–3.52		0.211
Mean ± S.D.	1.12 ± 0.66		1.26 ± 0.71		
FMC-to-N (min)					
Range	15–85		60.0–280		0.001 *
Mean ± S.D.	52.6 ± 22.8		125.0 ± 53.6		
	No.	%	No.	%	
MVD	43	11.8	63	23.3	0.389
SVD	321	88.2	207	76.7	
Culprit vessel					
LAD	216	59.3	128	47.4	
RCA	108	29.7	97	35.9	0.089
LCX	40	11	45	16.7	
Clopidogrel	221	60.7	155	57.3	0.410
Ticagrelor	143	39.3	115	42.7	

p value for comparing between the two studied groups. *: Statistically significant at $p \leq 0.05$.

3.2. Laboratory Findings

The incidence of lymphopenia was significantly higher in group B than in group A (14.78 ± 5.85 vs. 18.6 ± 6.21, $p = 0.012$), serum ferritin and D-dimer levels were also higher in group B than in group A. Cardiac enzymes, haemoglobin and serum creatinine did not differ between groups. The laboratory findings of both groups are shown in Table 1.

3.3. Time FMC-To-N

Patients in group B had significantly longer FMC-to-N compared to patients in group A (125.0 ± 53.6 vs. 52.6 ± 22.8, $p = 0.001$). The FMC-to-N of both groups is presented in Table 1.

3.4. Procedural Characteristics of the Two Groups

With regard to the angiographic data, the incidence of multivessel disease was not different between the two groups, as was the culprit artery. Also, the antiplatelet treatment with clopidogrel or ticagrelor did not differ. None of the patients in the two groups received fibrinolytic therapy. All patients in the two groups received drug eluting stents (DES) and no patient had procedure related dissection or perforation. The final TIMI flow at the end of the procedure was similar among patients of both groups. All patients received in-hospital medical treatment and follow up according to the latest STEMI guidelines [1,16]. Data of the procedural characteristics of the studied population are summarized in Table 1.

3.5. In-Hospital Outcomes

In hospital mortality was higher in group B (7.4 vs. 4.6%, $p = 0.036$) as was the incidence of re-infarction (12.2 vs. 7.7%) compared to group A, the difference between the two was significant ($p = 0.041$). Twenty patients in group B died, mostly because of arrhythmia (ventricular fibrillation) and the rest developed intractable cardiogenic shock and pulmonary edema. The need for revascularization was also higher in Group B (15.9 vs. 10.7%, $p = 0.046$) but the incidence of heart failure or bleeding was not different between groups. Although there was statistically high stroke prevalence in group A, we are unable to ascertain an exact explanation for it. One possible practice-based explanation for this finding is that in 2019 we used more thrombus aspiration catheters during PPCI than in 2020. The data of procedural outcomes are summarized in Table 2.

Table 2. In hospital outcomes of the studied population.

	Group A $n = 364$		Group B $n = 270$		p-Value
	No.	%	No.	%	
In-hospital mortality	17	4.6	20	7.4	0.036 *
Re-infarction	28	7.7	33	12.2	0.041 *
Need for revascularization	39	10.7	43	15.9	0.046 *
Heart Failure	117	32.1	96	35.6	0.258
CVS	20	5.5	10	3.7	0.022
Bleeding	39	10.7	30	11.1	0.511

p value for comparing between the two studied groups. *: Statistically significant at $p \leq 0.05$.

3.6. Duration of Hospitalization

The duration of hospital stay was significantly longer in group B compared with group A (6.85 ± 4.22 vs. 3.5 ± 2.3 day, $p = 0.0025$).

4. Discussion

Findings: COVID-19 pandemic has adversely affected various aspects of health care services including patients with heart disease and acute coronary syndrome [4]. The objective of this study was to evaluate the impact of COVID-19 on STEMI patients requiring conventional PPCI treatment and their clinical outcomes. Our results show that all studied

STEMI patients were treated with PPCI without need for fibrinolytic therapy, even for highly suspected COVID-19 patients. However, the frequency of PPCI treatment was significantly reduced and the intervention was delayed when compared with 2019 controls. Also, the hospital stay was prolonged and associated with some complications including re-infarction, need for coronary artery bypass surgery, CVS and increased in-hospital mortality. Despite that, the prevalence of developed heart failure and bleeding was not different from controls, treated by similar strategy a year before COVID-19.

Comparative results: Our findings can be summarized in showing significant change in STEMI practice during COVID-19 with delayed acute presentation and its management. The delay in presentation was mainly due to patients' fear of catching the viral infection at the hospital. This finding in ICC is compatible with other countries. HunShing Kwok et al. reported a dramatic reduction in PPCI procedures in the UK during the lockdown period [18], Dingcheng Xiang et al. reported 62% less PPCI in China [19], and 73 centers reported 40% reduction in PPCI in Spain [20]. The delayed PPCI was merely due to the screening tests performed before procedure, particularly in highly suspected patients who occasionally required other necessary investigations first, e.g., chest computed tomography (CT) scans. The increased in-hospital mortality with COVID-19 is similar to that reported by Dingcheng Xiang et al. [19] but contradicted Hun Shing Kwok et al. reports [18]. Other important findings in our study were the increased rate of re-infarction, the need for revascularization and the doubled hospital stay period, during the pandemic despite similar incidence of heart failure, stroke and bleeding. These findings were similar to that reported by Dingcheng Xiang et al. [19] but contradicted Hun Shing Kwok et al. results [18] which reported significant reduction ofin-hospital stay period.

It seems therefore that the internationally agreed impact of COVID-19 on conventional interventional management of STEMI is mainly during the acute phase of the disease with delayed presentation, reduced number of cases, and delayed procedure. While the former is mainly patient related, the latter is hospital controlled which is based on the nature of presentation of individual patients. In this scenario, it cannot be ignored that the rest of the clinical outcome is determined by the extent of co-morbidities, and severity of COVID-19 infection which vary between individual patients.

Limitations: This study has some obvious limitations. The recruited patients were those referred to the ICC hospital with STEMI diagnosis, mostly by individual cardiologists or other local hospitals, thus do not reflect a population. The follow-up duration was short and concerned only in-hospital stay, based on the study nature and design. Although patients were referred from different sources, they were all managed in one center from which the results were generated.

5. Conclusions

Our study shows that COVID-19 was associated with a significant decrease in the number of STEMI patients treated by PPCI at the ICC- Egypt, delayed procedure, higher in-hospital mortality, higher rates of re-infarction, need for repeat revascularization, and longer duration of hospital stay but with similar rates of heart failure, stroke, and bleeding.

Author Contributions: Conceptualization, S.A., R.S., and M.H.; Methodology, S.A., M.H., and R.S.; Software, R.S.; Validation, S.A.; Formal analysis, S.A., R.S., and M.H.; Investigation, S.A., M.H., and R.S.; Writing—original draft preparation, S.A.; Writing—review and editing, S.A., M.H., and R.S. All authors have read and agreed to the published version of the manuscript.

Funding: This research received no external funding.

Institutional Review Board Statement: The study was conducted according to the guidelines of the Declaration of Helsinki, and approved by Faculty of Medicine, Alexandria University Ethics Committee. (Approval number 0304893-Approval date 19/11/20).

Informed Consent Statement: Informed consent was obtained from all subjects involved in the study.

Data Availability Statement: Data available in a publicly accessible repository.

Conflicts of Interest: The authors declare no conflict of interest.

Abbreviations

CABG: coronary artery bypass grafting; LCX: left circumflex artery; STEMI: ST segment elevation myocardial infarction; PPCI: primary percutaneous coronary intervention; TIMI: Thrombolysis In Myocardial Infarction; MACCE: Major Adverse Cardiac and Cerebrovascular Events; CVS: cerebrovascular stroke; RCA: right coronary artery; LAD: left anterior descending artery; LM: left main; MVD: multi-vessel disease; SVD: single vessel disease; TVR: target vessel revascularization; FMC-to-N: first medical contact to needle time;COVID-19: corona virus disease-2019; WHO: world health organization; DES: drug eluting stents; ICC: International Cardiac Center; CK-MB: creatinine kinase—MB isoenzyme.

References

1. Ibanez, B.; James, S.; Agewall, S.; Antunes, M.J.; Bucciarelli-Ducci, C.; Bueno, H.; Caforio, A.L.P.; Crea, F.; Goudevenos, J.A.; Halvorsen, S.; et al. 2017 ESC Guidelines for the management of acute myocardial infarction in patients presenting with ST-segment elevation: The Task Force for the management of acute myocardial infarction in patients presenting with ST-segment elevation of the European Society of Cardiology (ESC). *Eur. Heart J.* **2018**, *39*, 119–177. [PubMed]
2. Guerchicoff, A.; Brener, S.J.; Maehara, A.; Witzenbichler, B.; Fahy, M.; Xu, K.; Gersh, B.J.; Mehran, R.; Gibson, C.M.; Stone, G.W. Impact of delay to reperfusion on reperfusion success, infarct size, and clinical outcomes in patients with ST-segment elevation myocardial infarction: The INFUSE-AMI trial (INFUSE-anterior myocardial infarction). *JACC Cardiovasc. Interv.* **2014**, *7*, 733–740. [CrossRef] [PubMed]
3. Nallamothu, B.K.; Normand, S.-L.T.; Wang, Y.; Hofer, T.P.; Brush, J.E.; Messenger, J.C.; Bradley, E.H.; Rumsfeld, J.S.; Krumholz, H.M. Relation between door-to-balloon times and mortality after primary percutaneous coronary intervention over time: A retrospective study. *Lancet* **2015**, *385*, 1114–1122. [CrossRef]
4. WHO. Clinical management of severe acute respiratory infection (SARI) when COVID-19 disease is suspected. Interim guidance. *Pediatr. Med. Rodz.* **2020**, *16*, 9–26. Available online: https://www.researchgate.net/publication/342941087_Clinical_management_of_severe_acute_respiratory_infection_SARI_when_COVID-19_disease_is_suspected_Interim_guidance (accessed on 13 March 2020). [CrossRef]
5. Daralammouri, Y.; Azamtta, M.; Hamayel, H.; Jaber, D.A.; Adas, A.; Hussein, I.-E.; Hantash, H.A.; Hammoudeh, A.; Mousa, E.; Nasr, M. Recommendations for safe and effective practice of interventional cardiology during COVID-19 pandemic: Expert opinion from Jordan and Palestine. *Palest. Med. Pharm. J.* **2020**, *5*, 65–73.
6. Xiang, D.; Huo, Y.; Ge, J. Expert consensus on operating procedures at chest pain centers in China during the coronavirus infec-tious disease-19 epidemic. *Cardiol. Plus* **2020**, *5*, 21–32. [CrossRef]
7. Sadeghipour, P.; Talasaz, A.H.; Eslami, V.; Geraiely, B.; Vojdanparast, M.; Sedaghat, M.; Moosavi, A.F.; Alipour-Parsa, S.; Aminian, B.; Firouzi, A.; et al. Management of ST-segment-elevation myocardial infarction during the coronavirus disease 2019 (COVID-19) outbreak: Iranian "247" National Committee's position paper on primary percutaneous coronary intervention. *Catheter. Cardiovasc. Interv.* **2020**. [CrossRef]
8. Szerlip, M.; Anwaruddin, S.; Aronow, H.D.; Cohen, M.G.; Daniels, M.J.; Dehghani, P.; Drachman, D.E.; Elmariah, S.; Feldman, D.N.; Garcia, S.; et al. Considerations for cardiac catheterization laboratory procedures during the COVID-19 pandemic. *Catheter. Cardiovasc. Interv.* **2020**, *96*, 586–597. [CrossRef]
9. Zaman, S.; MacIsaac, A.I.; Jennings, G.L.; Schlaich, M.P.; Inglis, S.C.; Arnold, R.; Kumar, S.; Thomas, L.; Wahi, S.; Lo, S.; et al. Cardiovascular disease and COVID-19: Australian and New Zealand consensus statement. *Med. J. Aust.* **2020**, *213*, 182–187. [CrossRef]
10. Uccio, F.S.D.; Valente, S.; Colivicchi, F.; Murrone, A.; Caldarola, P.; Lenarda, A.D.; Roncon, L.; Amodeo, E.; Aspromonte, N.; Cipriani, M.G.; et al. ANMCO position paper: The network organization for the management of patients with acute coronary syndrome during the COVID-19 pandemic. *Eur. Heart J.* **2020**, *21*, 332–335.
11. Mahmud, E.; Dauerman, H.L.; Welt, F.G.; Messenger, J.C.; Rao, S.V.; Grines, C.; Mattu, A.; Kirtane, A.J.; Jauhar, R.; Meraj, P.; et al. Management of acute myocardial infarction during the COVID-19 pandemic: A position statement from the Society for Cardiovascular Angiography and Interventions (SCAI), the American College of Cardiology (ACC), and the American College of Emergency Physicians (ACEP). *J. Am. Coll. Cardiol.* **2020**, *76*, 1375–1384. [PubMed]
12. Garcia, S.; Albaghdadi, M.S.; Meraj, P.M.; Schmidt, C.; Garberich, R.; Jaffer, F.A.; Dixon, S.; Rade, J.J.; Tannenbaum, M.; Chambers, J.; et al. Reduction in ST-segment elevation cardiac catheterization laboratory activations in the United States during COVID-19 pandemic. *J. Am. Coll. Cardiol.* **2020**, *75*, 2871–2872. [CrossRef] [PubMed]
13. De Rosa, S.; Spaccarotella, C.; Basso, C.; Calabro, A.C.; Filardi, P.P.; Mancone, M.; Mercuri, G.; Muscoli, S.; Nodari, S.; Pedrinelli, R.; et al. Reduction of hospitalizations for myocardial infarction in Italy in the COVID-19 era. *Eur. Heart J.* **2020**, *41*, 2083–2088. [PubMed]

14. Tam, C.-C.F.; Cheung, K.-S.; Lam, S.; Wong, A.; Yung, A.; Sze, M.; Lam, Y.-M.; Chan, C.; Tsang, T.-C.; Tsui, M.; et al. Impact of Coronavirus Disease 2019 (COVID-19) Outbreak on ST-Segment–Elevation Myocardial Infarction Care in Hong Kong, China. *Circ. Cardiovasc. Qual. Outcomes* **2020**, *13*, e006631. [CrossRef] [PubMed]
15. Ranard, L.S.; Ahmad, Y.; Masoumi, A.; Chuich, T.; Romney, M.-L.S.; Gavin, N.; Sayan, O.R.; Kirtane, A.J.; Rabbani, L.E. Clinical Pathway for Management of Suspected or Positive Novel Coronavirus-19 Patients With ST-Segment Elevation Myocardial Infarction. *Crit. Pathw. Cardiol.* **2020**, *19*, 49–54. [CrossRef] [PubMed]
16. Thygesen, K.; Alpert, J.S.; Jaffe, A.S.; Chaitman, B.R.; Bax, J.J.; Morrow, D.A.; White, H.D. Fourth Universal Definition of Myocardial Infarction (2018). *Circulation* **2018**, *138*, e618–e651. [CrossRef] [PubMed]
17. Kirkpatrick, L.A.; Feeney, B.C. *A Simple Guide to IBM SPSS Statistics for Version 20.0*, Student ed.; Wadsworth, Cengage Learning: Belmont, CA, USA, 2013.
18. Kwok, C.S.; Gale, C.P.; Kinnaird, T.; Curzen, N.; Ludman, P.; Kontopantelis, E.; Wu, J.; Denwood, T.; Fazal, N.; Deanfield, J.; et al. Impact of COVID-19 on percutaneous coronary intervention for ST-elevation myocardial infarction. *Heart* **2020**, *106*, 1805–1811. [CrossRef] [PubMed]
19. Xiang, D.; Xiang, X.; Zhang, W.; Yi, S.; Zhang, J.; Gu, X.; Xu, Y.; Huang, K.; Su, X.; Yu, B.; et al. Management and Outcomes of Patients with STEMI During the COVID-19 Pandemic in China. *J. Am. Coll. Cardiol.* **2020**, *76*, 1318–1324. [CrossRef] [PubMed]
20. Rodríguez-Leor, O.; Cid-Álvarez, B.; Ojeda, S.; Martín-Moreiras, J.; Rumoroso, J.R.; López-Palop, R.; Serrador, A.; Cequier, Á.; Romaguera, R.; Cruz, I.; et al. Impact of the COVID-19 pandemic on interventional cardiology activity in Spain. *REC Interv. Cardiol.* **2020**, *2*, 82–89. [CrossRef]

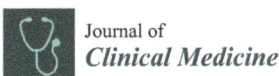

Article

Combined Cardiac Risk Factors Predict COVID-19 Related Mortality and the Need for Mechanical Ventilation in Coptic Clergy

Michael Y. Henein [1,2,3,*,†], Ibadete Bytyçi [1,†], Rachel Nicoll [1], Rafik Shenouda [1,4], Sherif Ayad [5], Matteo Cameli [6] and Federico Vancheri [7]

1. Institute of Public Health and Clinical Medicine, Umea University, 90187 Umea, Sweden; i.bytyci@hotmail.com (I.B.); rachelnicoll25@gmail.com (R.N.); rafik.sheneuda@umu.se (R.S.)
2. Molecular and Clinic Research Institute, St George University, London SW17 0QT, UK
3. Institute of Fluid Dynamics, Brunel University, London UB8 3PH, UK
4. International Cardiac Centre, Alexandria 21526, Egypt
5. Department of Cardiology, Faculty of Medicine, Alexandria University, Alexandria 21526, Egypt; sherifwagdyayad@yahoo.com
6. Department of Cardiovascular Disease, University of Siena, 53100 Siena, Italy; matteo.cameli@yahoo.com
7. Department of Internal Medicine, S. Elia Hospital, 93100 Caltanissetta, Italy; federico.vancheri@ki.se
* Correspondence: michael.henein@umu.se; Tel.: +46-90-785-14-31
† Michael Y. Henein and Ibadete Bytyçi contributed equally.

Abstract: Background and Aims: The clinical adverse events of COVID-19 among clergy worldwide have been found to be higher than among ordinary communities, probably because of the nature of their work. The aim of this study was to assess the impact of cardiac risk factors on COVID-19-related mortality and the need for mechanical ventilation in Coptic clergy. Methods: Of 1570 Coptic clergy participating in the COVID-19-Clergy study, serving in Egypt, USA and Europe, 213 had the infection and were included in this analysis. Based on the presence of systemic arterial hypertension (AH), participants were divided into two groups: Group-I, clergy with AH ($n = 77$) and Group-II, without AH ($n = 136$). Participants' demographic indices, cardiovascular risk factors, COVID-19 management details and related mortality were assessed. Results: Clergy with AH were older ($p < 0.001$), more obese ($p = 0.04$), had frequent type 2 diabetes (DM) ($p = 0.001$), dyslipidemia ($p = 0.001$) and coronary heart disease (CHD) ($p = 0.04$) compared to those without AH. COVID-19 treatment at home, hospital or in intensive care did not differ between the patient groups ($p > 0.05$ for all). Clergy serving in Northern and Southern Egypt had a higher mortality rate compared to those from Europe and the USA combined (5.22%, 6.38%, 0%; $p = 0.001$). The impact of AH on mortality was significant only in Southern Egypt (10% vs. 3.7%; $p = 0.01$) but not in Northern Egypt (4.88% vs. 5.81%; $p = 0.43$). In multivariate analysis, CHD OR 1.607 ((0.982 to 3.051); $p = 0.02$) and obesity, OR 3.403 ((1.902 to 4.694); $p = 0.04$) predicted COVID-19 related mortality. A model combining cardiac risk factors (systolic blood pressure (SBP) ≥ 160 mmHg, DM, obesity and history of CHD) was the most powerful independent predictor of COVID-19-related mortality, OR 3.991 ((1.919 to 6.844); $p = 0.002$). Almost the same model also proved the best independent multivariate predictor of mechanical ventilation OR 1.501 ((0.809 to 6.108); $p = 0.001$). Conclusion: In Coptic clergy, the cumulative impact of risk factors was the most powerful predictor of mortality and the need for mechanical ventilation.

Keywords: COVID-19; Coptic clergy; mortality; cardiovascular risk factors

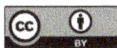

1. Introduction

COVID-19 is an aggressive pandemic that has claimed the lives of millions worldwide [1], and many of those recovering may develop serious long-term symptoms. First wave studies [2,3] reported a higher mortality rate among the black, Asian and minority ethnic (BAME) communities, highlighting the importance of ethnic impact on the natural history of the disease. In addition, most sufferers requiring mechanical ventilation have been found to have significant co-morbidities [4]. On the other hand, social distancing has played an important role in controlling, to a great extent, the rate of disease transmission with its associated mortality [5,6], and vaccination has provided significant protection, particularly among the elderly [7,8].

We have previously reported high COVID-19 prevalence among Coptic clergy and explained it on the basis of their lifestyle and regular community service, which requires close contact with their parishioners. We have also highlighted the important role of obesity in explaining this high disease prevalence [9]. The aim of this study is to assess the additional role of conventional cardiovascular risk factors in predicting mortality and the need for mechanical ventilation in Coptic clergy with COVID-19.

2. Methods

2.1. Study Design and Patients

The present study is a retrospective evaluation of a cohort of 1576 Coptic clergy worldwide, from March to December 2020. It is a sub-study within the COVID-19-CVD international study, which is investigating the impact of COVID-19 on the cardiovascular system and which has been approved by the Swedish Ethics Board (Dnr 2020-02217 Stockholm avdelning 2 medicin). M.Y.H. (The principal investigator) designed the study protocol which was endorsed by the Head of the Coptic Church in Egypt. 1570 clergy within 25 dioceses were evaluated from different areas of Egypt, Europe and the USA. Dioceses in Egypt were divided into two main regions, Northern (comprising Alexandria, the Delta and Cairo) and Southern (comprising all cities geographically south of Cairo). Data collected from Coptic clergy serving in the European countries and the USA were combined and analyzed as one group since they mostly follow similar disease prevention and treatment strategies. According to the presence of arterial hypertension (AH), the clergy suffering COVID-19 were divided into two groups: Group-I: clergy with AH (n = 77) and Group-II: clergy without AH (n = 136). 13 infected clergy were excluded due to lack of clinical data (Figure 1).

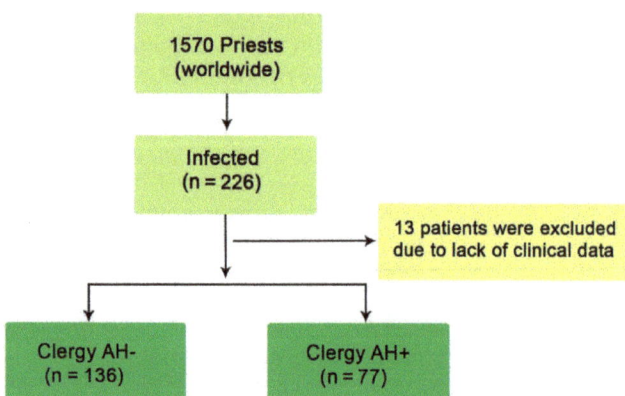

Figure 1. Flow chart of participants.

2.2. Cardiovascular Risk Factor Assessment

Cardiovascular risk factors such as arterial hypertension (AH), type 2 diabetes mellitus (DM), coronary heart disease (CHD), dyslipidemia, obesity and family history of cardiovascular disease were assessed based on medical records and prior investigations and management. According to conventional international risk factor assessment and cut-off values for body mass index (BMI), overweight was defined as BMI of 25–29.9 kg/m^2 and obesity as BMI $\geq$30 kg/m^2. Systemic AH was diagnosed when systolic blood pressure (SBP) was $\geq$130 mmHg and/or diastolic blood pressure (DBP) was $\geq$80 mmHg. Type

2 diabetes mellitus (DM) was identified based on pre-recruitment diagnosis leading to participants commenced on conventional oral hypoglycemics and/or insulin therapy. Dyslipidemia was determined from medical records or if the individual had been commenced on statins. Evidence for coronary artery disease was also evaluated from medical records, based on prior investigations and management.

2.3. Clinical Events

Clinical events (CE) were retrospectively collected and information on participants' clinical outcome was obtained from electronic medical records, clinical visits, personal communication with general physicians and confidential telephone interviews with patients and relatives. The study's primary outcome was COVID-19-related mortality; the secondary outcome was the need for mechanical ventilation.

2.4. Statistical Analysis

Discrete data are reported as frequencies (percentages) and continuous variables are shown as means and standard deviation (SD) if normally distributed, or median and interquartile range (IQR: Q1–Q3) in case of skewed distribution. Continuous data were compared with the two-tailed Student t-test and discrete data with Chi-square test. Analysis of variance and Bonferroni statistical tests were used to compare quantitative variables between more than two groups. Predictors of mortality related to COVID-19 and the need for mechanical ventilation were identified with univariate analysis. Independent predictors were identified using multivariate logistic regression analysis using the stepwise method. A significant difference was defined as p-value < 0.05 (two-tailed). Statistical analysis was performed with SPSS Software Package version 26.0 (IBM Corp., Armonk, NY, USA).

3. Results

3.1. Demographic and Clinical Indices for Clergy with COVID-19

Two hundred and thirteen symptomatic clergy with COVID-19 were included in the study. Patients' mean age was 49.6 ± 12 years and all were males. Out of the 213 clergy, 122 (57.3%) were obese, 59 (27.7%) had diabetes, 68 (31.9%) had dyslipidemia and 20 (9.4%) had coronary artery disease. 171/213 (80.2%) of the clergy were treated at home and the remaining 26 (16.9%) in hospital, 17 (7.9%) of them needed intensive care management and 15 (7.1%) required mechanical ventilation (Tables 1 and 2).

Table 1. Demographic and clinical data between clergy groups.

Variable	Clergy	Clergy AH-	Clergy AH+	p
	(n = 213)	(n = 136)	(n = 77)	Value
Demographic and Clinical Data				
Age (years)	49.6 ± 12	46.3 ± 11	56.1 ± 11	<0.001
BMI (m/kg^2)	31.9 ± 6.2	31.5 ± 6.3	33.1 ± 5.9	0.09
SBP (mmHg)	127 ± 13	121 ± 8.5	135 ± 14	<0.001
DBP (mmHg)	83 ± 9.1	81 ± 6.6	87 ± 11	<0.001
Underweight (n, %)	0 (0)	0 (0)	0 (0)	0.91
Normal weight (n, %)	17 (7.9)	12 (9.3)	5 (6.3)	0.12
Overweight (n, %)	74 (34.7)	54 (39.7)	20 (15.5)	0.02
Obese (n, %)	122 (57.3)	70 (51.7)	52 (68.2)	0.04
DM (n, %)	59 (27.7)	26 (19.1)	33 (43.2)	0.001
Dyslipidemia	68 (31.9)	22 (16.4)	46 (60.6)	0.001
CHD (n, %)	20 (9.4)	10 (7.4)	10 (13.6)	0.04
Family history of CHD (n, %)	22 (10.3)	10 (7.4)	12 (15.6)	0.01
Family history of stroke (n, %)	16 (7.5)	6 (4.76)	10 (10.3)	0.04

AH+, with arterial hypertension; AH-, without arterial hypertension; BMI, body mass index; CHD, coronary heart disease; DM, diabetes mellitus; SBP, systolic blood pressure; DBP, diastolic blood pressure.

Table 2. Outcome data between clergy groups.

Variable	Clergy	Clergy AH-	Clergy AH+	p
	(n = 213)	(n = 136)	(n = 77)	Value
Outcome data				
Home treatment (n, %)	171 (80.2)	110 (81.6)	61 (78.7)	0.55
Hospital treatment (n, %)	36 (16.9)	21 (15.4)	15 (19.7)	0.23
Intensive care (n, %)	17 (7.9)	11 (8.3)	6 (8.3)	0.81
Prevalence (%)	13.6	10.2	20.1	0.001
Mechanical ventilator (n, %)	15 (7.1)	8 (5.9)	7 (9.1)	0.09
Death (n, %)	10 (4.69)	5 (3.68)	5 (6.49)	0.058

AH+, with arterial hypertension; AH-, without arterial hypertension.

3.2. Demographic and Clinical Data of Clergy with and without AH

Compared to clergy without AH, the prevalence of COVID-19 was higher in those with AH (20.1% vs. 10.2%). Clergy with AH were older ($p < 0.001$), more obese ($p = 0.04$), had more diabetes ($p = 0.001$), dyslipidemia ($p = 0.001$) and coronary heart disease (CHD) ($p = 0.04$) compared to those without AH. Family history for cardiovascular disease, stroke or CHD did not differ between patient groups ($p > 0.05$ for both). The frequency of management at home, hospital or intensive care did not differ between patient groups with or without AH ($p > 0.05$ for all, Table 1).

3.3. Geographical Impact on Clinical Events

Among the 213 clergy with COVID-19, the overall mortality rate was 4.69% and the need for mechanical ventilation was 7.1% (Table 2). Based on geographical analysis, the overall clergy mortality rate in Northern (n = 136, 51 with AH) and Southern Egypt (n = 46; 14 with AH) was higher compared to that in Europe and USA combined (5.22%, 6.51%, 0%, respectively; $p = 0.001$). The impact of AH on mortality was not significant in Northern (5.88% vs. 4.71%, respectively; $p = 0.22$) and Southern Egypt (7.1% vs. 6.21%, respectively; $p = 0.43$) compared to those without AH (Table 3).

Table 3. Geographical impact on clinical outcome.

Variable	EU +USA	Northern Egypt	Southern Egypt	p
	(n = 31)	(n = 136)	(n = 46)	Value
Death (n, %)	0 (0)	7 (5.22) [a,b]	3 (6.51) [a,b]	0.001
Clergy AH-	0 (0%)	4 (4.71)	2 (6.21) [a,b]	0.01
Clergy AH+	0 (0%)	3 (5.88)	1 (7.10) [a,b]	0.02

[a] $p < 0.05$; Gr. I vs. II [b] $p < 0.05$; Gr. I vs. III [c] $p < 0.05$; Gr. II vs. III. AH+, with arterial hypertension; AH-, without arterial hypertension.

3.4. Distribution of Cardiac Risk Factors among Clergy with and without Adverse Clinical Events

The overall mortality rate in the study participants was 4.69% with no difference between clergy with and without AH (4.41% vs. 5.19% $p = 0.12$). The prevalence of risk factors among the deceased clergy compared to survivors were: CHD (44.4% vs. 7.81%; $p = 0.001$), obesity (78.1 vs. 45.1%, $p < 0.001$), and AH trends to be more prevalent (35.6% vs. 30.2%; $p = 0.052$), but DM (22.2% vs. 23.7%; $p = 0.44$), and dyslipidemia (33.1% vs. 31.1%; $p = 0.18$) were not different. However, the combined cardiac risk factors (AH, CHD, DM, obesity and dyslipidemia) were more prevalent among deceased clergy compared to survivors (33% vs. 7.56%; $p < 0.001$ Figure 2). Likewise, combined risk factors were more prevalent in the 15 (7.1%) clergy requiring mechanical ventilation compared to those who did not (20% vs. 7.27%; $p < 0.001$) (Figure 3).

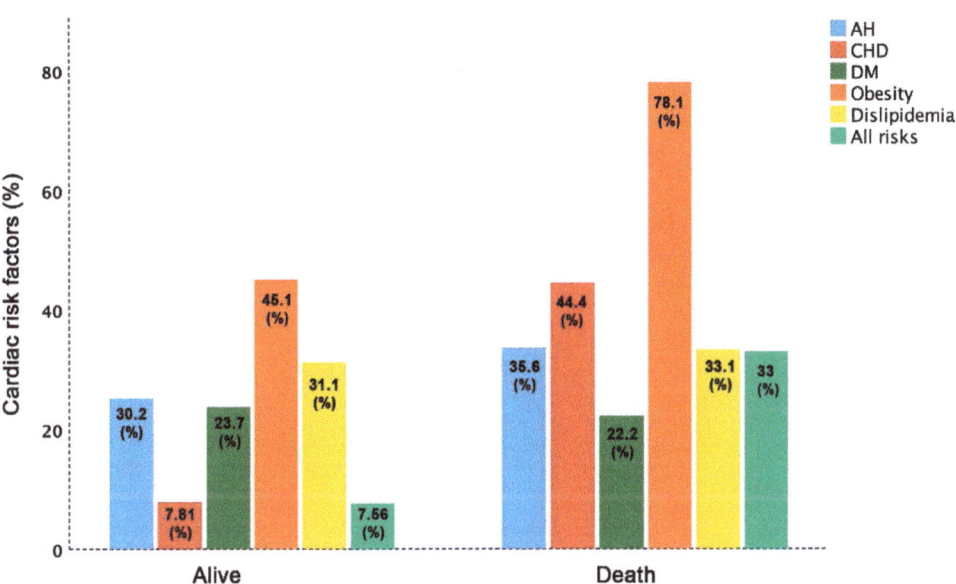

Figure 2. Distribution of cardiac risk factors among living and deceased clergy.

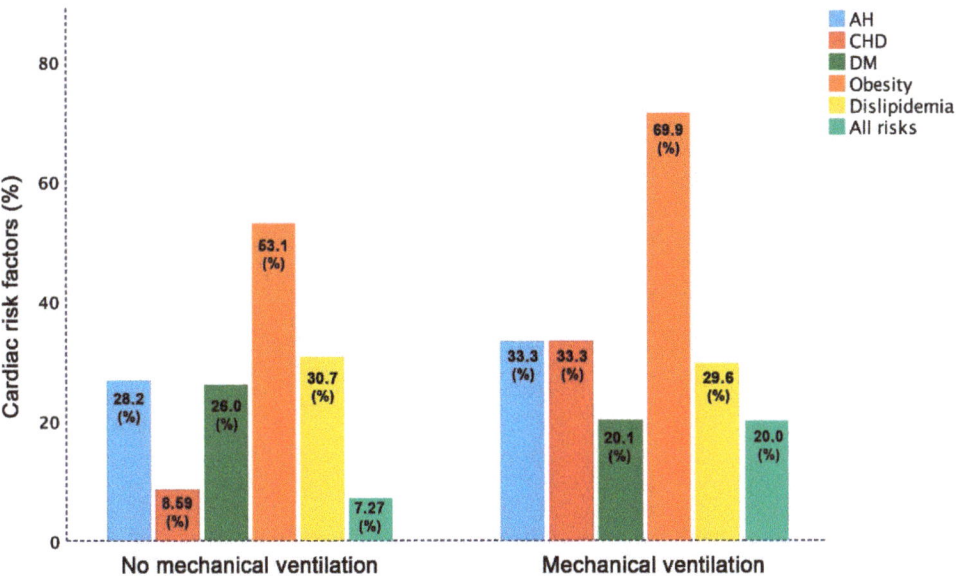

Figure 3. Distribution of cardiac risk factors among clergy based on the need for mechanical ventilation.

3.5. Predictors of COVID-19-Related Adverse Clinical Events

Mortality prediction: In univariate analysis, DM (p = 0.02), obesity (p = 0.03), AH (0.04) and CHD (p = 0.001) predicted COVID-19-related mortality. In multivariate analysis, only CHD (OR 1.607 ((0.982 to 3.051); p = 0.02)) and obesity (OR 3.403 ((1.902 to 4.694; p = 0.04)) predicted mortality. A model combining cardiac risk factors including: SBP $\geq$160 mmHg, DM, obesity and CHD proved the most powerful independent predictor of mortality (OR 3.991 ((1.919 to 6.844); p = 0.002) (Table 4).

Table 4. Predictors of mortality and mechanical ventilation in COVID-19 patients.

Variable	Univariate Predictors	p	Multivariate Predictors	p
	OR (95% CI)	Value	OR (95% CI)	Value
	Mortality			
Diabetes	0.845 (0.045 to 2.896)	0.02	1.003 (0.202 to 3.804)	0.09
Obesity	2.301 (1.002 to 4.094)	0.03	3.403 (1.902 to 4.694)	0.04
AH	0.918 (0.103 to 2.191)	0.04	1.403 (0.802 to 4.001)	0.23
Dyslipidemia	1.031 (0.007 to 4.019)	0.11	2.003 (1.002 to 4.309)	0.33
CHD	1.219 (1.098 to 3.004)	0.001	1.607 (0.982 to 3.051)	0.02
Family history for CHD	0.605 (0.025 to 4.106)	0.21		
Family history for stroke	0.729 (0.171 to 2.649)	0.42		
Diabetes	0.845 (0.045 to 2.896)	0.02	0.146 (0.013 to 1.189)	0.08
Obesity	2.301 (1.002 to 4.094)	0.03	3.174 (0.254 to 9.679)	0.31
AH	0.918 (0.103 to 2.191)	0.04	0.587 (0.003 to 5.191)	0.63
Dyslipidemia	1.031 (0.007 to 4.019)	0.11	0.707 (0.101 to 4.201)	0.63
CHD	1.219 (1.098 to 3.004)	0.001	0.936 (1.082 to 8.517)	0.86
Model *	2.400 (0.509 to 1.400)	0.001	3.991 (1.919 to 6.844)	0.002
	Mechanical ventilation			
Diabetes	0.641 (0.077 to 3.377)	0.51	0.641 (0.077 to 3.377)	0.63
Obesity	3.872 (1.771 to 10.72)	0.01	3.872 (1.771 to 10.72)	0.01
AH	2.347 (1.197 to 4.501)	0.03	2.347 (1.197 to 4.501)	0.23
Dyslipidemia	1.056 (0.310 to 3.594)	0.87	1.056 (0.310 to 3.594)	0.77
CHD	5.321 (1.410 to 9.908)	0.01	5.321 (1.410 to 9.908)	0.01
Diabetes	0.641 (0.077 to 3.377)	0.51	0.209 (0.027 to 1.616)	0.13
Obesity	3.872 (1.771 to 10.72)	0.01	1.358 (0.273 to 6.748)	0.27
AH	2.347 (1.197 to 4.501)	0.03	0.067 (0.007 to 1.145)	0.06
Dyslipidemia	1.056 (0.310 to 3.594)	0.87	0.098 (0.010 to 7.104)	0.81
CHD	5.321 (1.410 to 9.908)	0.01	3.235 (0.451 to 23.19)	0.24
Model **	1.807 (0.750 to 2.991)	<0.001	1.501 (0.809 to 6.108)	0.001

Model * (SBP ≥ 160 mmHg, DM+, Obesity+, CHD+); Model ** (SBP ≥ 160 mmHg, Obesity+, CHD+); AH, arterial hypertension; BMI, body mass index; CHD, Coronary heart disease; DM, diabetes mellitus; SBP, Systolic blood pressure; DBP, diastolic blood pressure.

Mechanical ventilation prediction: CHD (OR 5.321 (1.410 to 9.908)) and obesity (OR 3.872 ((1.771 to 10.72); p = 0.02)) predicted the need for mechanical ventilation in a multivariate analysis model. Almost the same model above, combining cardiac risk factors, proved the strongest independent multivariate predictor of the need for mechanical ventilation (OR 1.501 ((0.809 to 6.108); p = 0.001)) (Table 4). Collinearity between these measurements was not met based on VIF <10 for all predictors.

4. Discussion

Findings: The results of this cohort study reveal the following: (1) Cardiac risk factors were more prevalent among Coptic clergy with arterial hypertension (AH) compared to those without AH; (2) The mortality rate increased linearly with the increasing number of cardiac risk factors; (3) Clergy serving in Northern and Southern Egypt had a higher mortality rate compared to those in Europe and USA combined; (4) The impact of AH on mortality was significant only in Southern Egypt; (5) A model combining cardiac risk factors was the best independent multivariate predictor of COVID-19-related mortality and the need for mechanical ventilation.

Data interpretation: The Framingham study established the important relationship between atherosclerosis risk factors, namely hypertension, diabetes, dyslipidemia, obesity and smoking on cardiovascular disease, particularly coronary artery disease and acute events [10,11]. It has also established the significant benefit of optimum risk factor control on clinical outcome, including survival and acute events, e.g., myocardial infarction and stroke [12,13]. Moreover, at the beginning of 2020, the American College of Cardiology (ACC) proposed clinical guidance focused on the cardiac implication in COVID-19 and recommendations for the Centers for best Disease Control and Prevention [14]. Those recommendations were further strengthened by meta-analyses based on clinical trials, which led to the currently available clinical guidelines of disease prevention [15,16]. Coptic clergy should not be seen as different, based on the abundance of risk factors they carry, as we have previously demonstrated [9]. Obesity was found to be the most prevalent risk factor and the main predictor of the significantly high prevalence of COVID-19 among the Coptic clergy [9,17]. The impact of obesity on the immune system is already well established and explains this high prevalence of COVID-19 among the clergy.

Our current findings go on to highlight the importance of the many cardiac risk factors which may be found among Coptic clergy. This is likely to be related to their lifestyle, particularly the lack of exercise undertaken, as a result of the significantly high demands on their time [18]. However, we are hereby showing clearly that ignoring optimum control of those risk factors, particularly in clergy suffering from COVID-19, puts them at a significantly high risk of mortality and need for mechanical ventilation, with its known problems and uncertain clinical outcome. These findings highlight the serious need for optimum risk factor control, lifestyle improvement and active immune system support. Perhaps a well-designed and balanced education program for Coptic clergy should be devised in different local languages, with recommendations for strict adherence to guidelines. Such a strategy, if seriously and religiously implemented, could only result in improved clinical outcomes.

Clinical implications: Coptic clergy suffering from COVID-19 are at high risk of mortality and need for mechanical ventilation if admitted to intensive care units. This health hazard can be strongly predicted by their cumulative cardiovascular risk factors. Since most risk factors are controllable, a strict education program should assist the clergy in avoiding this risk and in implementing a healthy lifestyle, leading to a stronger immune system.

Severe Covid-19 is often characterized by a dysregulated immune response, leading to lymphopenia and the cytokine storm, which attacks healthy tissue and is often fatal. Excessive cytokine production and their sustained elevation were found to provide a "core" COVID-19 signature; some of these cytokines are associated with blood clotting, another common concern in severe COVID-19. [19] A recent meta-analysis showed that in older patients, hypertension, diabetes and cardiovascular disease, all known inflammatory conditions, conveyed a higher risk of severe COVID-19 and/or mortality, with ORs of 2.5, 2.25 and 3.11, respectively. [20] Obesity, another inflammatory condition, is also a key risk factor for severe COVID-19 and has been shown to weaken the immune system by expanding adipose tissue production of pro-inflammatory cytokines and downregulating anti-inflammatory immune cells such as M2 macrophages, T helper (Th2) cells and regulatory T cells. [21,22] Similarly, in COVID-19 patients with hypertension, pre-activation of the immune cells has been found, manifesting as elevated inflammatory cytokines, which led to an augmented immune response in these patients on contact with the virus and delayed viral clearance [23]. In addition, angiotensin-converting enzyme 2 (ACE2) as aminopeptidase with key role in the cardiovascular and immune systems has been identified as a functional receptor for SARS-CoV2 by binding the spike protein of the virus to ACE2. It is highly expressed in the heart and lungs, particularly in alveolar epithelial cells in patients with COVID-19 and CVD and severe symptoms, in whom it might be associated with increased secretion of ACE2 compared to those without CVD [24].

Study limitations: The analyses undertaken in this study relied purely on the data received from the participants rather than direct control by the investigators. We designed the study and the information spreadsheet, which was sent to all dioceses, with a clear request to complete the data and send it to the principal investigator hence we have no hand in the data completion or accuracy. Not all Coptic dioceses contributed to the study, but there is no reason to suppose that the risk factors were materially different in other dioceses. Our suggestion concerning the expected impact of a specially devised education program remains to be tested and proved.

Conclusions: Coptic clergy carry multiple cardiovascular risk factors, which cumulatively are the most powerful predictors of COVID-19-related mortality and the need for mechanical ventilation.

Author Contributions: M.Y.H.: Conceptualization, study design, methodology and project administration; I.B.; R.S., S.A.; data sorting and statistical analysis; I.B., R.N., S.A., M.C., F.V.; data analysis and writing the first draft manuscript. All authors contributed to writing and approved the manuscript. All authors have read and agreed to the published version of the manuscript.

Funding: This research received no external funding.

Institutional Review Board Statement: Swedish Ethics Board (Dnr 2020-02217 Stockholm avdelning 2 medicin).

Informed Consent Statement: Informed consent was obtained from all subjects involved in the study.

Conflicts of Interest: The authors have no conflict of interest to declare.

References

1. Weiss, P.; Murdoch, D.R. Clinical course and mortality risk of severe COVID-19. *Lancet* **2020**, *395*, 1014–1015. [CrossRef]
2. Pillaye, J. Covid-19 and ethnic minorities: The Public Health England report distracts from proactive and timely intervention. *BMJ* **2020**, *370*, m3054. [CrossRef] [PubMed]
3. Keys, C.; Nanayakkara, G.; Onyejekwe, C.; Sah, R.K.; Wright, T. Health Inequalities and Ethnic Vulnerabilities During COVID-19 in the UK: A Reflection on the PHE Reports. *Fem. Leg. Stud.* **2021**, *14*, 1–12.
4. Shi, S.; Qin, M.; Shen, B.; Cai, Y.; Liu, T.; Yang, F.; Gong, W.; Liu, X.; Liang, J.; Zhao, Q.; et al. Association of Cardiac Injury With Mortality in Hospitalized Patients With COVID-19 in Wuhan, China. *JAMA Cardiol.* **2020**, *5*, 802–810. [CrossRef] [PubMed]
5. Chu, D.K.; Akl, E.A.; Duda, S.; Solo, K.; Yaacoub, S.; Schünemann, H.J.; COVID-19 Systematic Urgent Review Group Effort (SURGE) Study Authors. Physical distancing, face masks, and eye protection to prevent person-to-person transmission of SARS-CoV-2 and COVID-19: A systematic review and meta-analysis. *Lancet* **2020**, *395*, 1973–1987. [CrossRef]
6. WHO. Infection Prevention and Control during Health Care When Novel Coronavirus (nCoV) Infection Is Suspected. Interim Guidance. 2020. Available online: https://apps.who.int/iris/rest/bitstreams/1266296/retrieve (accessed on 1 March 2020).
7. Li, Y.D.; Chi, W.Y.; Su, J.H.; Ferrall, L.; Hung, C.F.; Wu, T.C. Coronavirus vaccine development: From SARS and MERS to COVID-19. *J. Biomed. Sci.* **2020**, *27*, 104. [CrossRef]
8. Izda, V.; Jeffries, M.A.; Sawalha, A.H. COVID-19: A review of therapeutic strategies and vaccine candidates. *Clin. Immunol.* **2021**, *222*, 108634. [CrossRef] [PubMed]
9. Henein, M.Y.; Bytyçi, I.; Nicoll, R.; Shenouda, R.; Ayad, S.; Vanchari, F.; Cameli, M. Obesity strongly predicts COVID-19-related major clinical adverse events in Coptic Clergy. 2021; submitted.
10. D'Agostino, R.B., Sr.; Pencina, M.J.; Massaro, J.M.; Coady, S. Cardiovascular Disease Risk Assessment: Insights from Framingham. *Glob. Heart* **2013**, *8*, 11–23. [CrossRef]
11. Kannel, W.B. Framingham study insights into hypertensive risk of cardiovascular disease. *Hypertens Res.* **1995**, *18*, 181–196. [CrossRef]
12. Wood, D.A.; Kotseva, K.; Connolly, S.; Jennings, C.; Mead, A.; Jones, J.; Holden, A.; de Bacquer, D.; Collier, T.; de Backer, G.; et al. Nurse-coordinated multidisciplinary, family-based cardiovascular disease prevention programme (EUROACTION) for patients with coronary heart disease and asymptomatic individuals at high risk of cardiovascular disease: A paired, cluster-randomised controlled trial. *Lancet* **2008**, *371*, 1999–2012.
13. Kones, R. Primary prevention of coronary heart disease: Integration of new data, evolving views, revised goals, and role of rosuvastatin in management. A comprehensive survey. *Drug Des. Dev. Ther.* **2011**, *5*, 325–380. [CrossRef]
14. Madjid, M.; Solomon, S.; Vardeny, O. ACC Clinical Bulletin: Cardiac Implications of Novel Wuhan Coronavirus (2019-nCoV). Available online: https://www.acc.org/latest-in-cardiology/articles/2020/02/13/12/42/acc-clinical-bulletin-focuses-on-cardiac-implications-of-coronavirus-2019-ncov (accessed on 13 February 2020).
15. Rozanski, A.; Bavishi, C.; Kubzansky, L.D.; Cohen, R. Association of Optimism with Cardiovascular Events and All-Cause Mortality: A Systematic Review and Meta-analysis. *JAMA Netw. Open* **2019**, *2*, e1912200. [CrossRef] [PubMed]
16. Arnett, D.K.; Blumenthal, R.S.; Albert, M.A.; Buroker, A.B.; Goldberger, Z.D.; Hahn, E.J.; Himmelfarb, C.D.; Khera, A.; Lloyd-Jones, D.; McEvoy, J.W.; et al. 2019 ACC/AHA Guideline on the Primary Prevention of Cardiovascular Disease: Executive Summary: A Report of the American College of Cardiology/American Heart Association Task Force on Clinical Practice Guidelines. *J. Am. Coll. Cardiol.* **2019**, *74*, 1376–1414. [CrossRef] [PubMed]
17. Ferguson, T.W.; Andercheck, B.; Tom, J.C.; Martinez, B.C.; Stroope, S. Occupational conditions, self-care, and obesity among clergy in the United States. *Soc. Sci. Res.* **2015**, *49*, 249–263. [CrossRef]
18. Proeschold-Bell, R.J.; LeGrand, S.H. High rates of obesity and chronic disease among United Methodist clergy. *Obesity* **2010**, *18*, 1867–1870. [CrossRef]

19. Lucas, C.; Team, Y.I.; Wong, P.; Klein, J.; Castro, T.B.R.; Silva, J.; Sundaram, M.; Ellingson, M.K.; Mao, T.; Oh, J.E.; et al. Longitudinal analyses reveal immunological misfiring in severe COVID-19. *Nature* **2020**, *584*, 463–469. [CrossRef]
20. Bae, S.; Kim, S.R.; Kim, M.; Shim, W.J.; Park, S.-M. Impact of cardiovascular disease and risk factors on fatal outcomes in patients with COVID-19 according to age: A systematic review and meta-analysis. *Heart* **2021**, *107*, 373–380. [CrossRef] [PubMed]
21. Chiappetta, S.; Sharma, A.M.; Bottino, V.; Stier, C. COVID-19 and the role of chronic inflammation in patients with obesity. *Int. J. Obes.* **2020**, *44*, 1790–1792. [CrossRef]
22. Mohammad, S.; Aziz, R.; Al Mahri, S.; Malik, S.S.; Haji, E.; Khan, A.H.; Khatlani, T.S.; Bouchama, A. Obesity and COVID-19: What makes obese host so vulnerable? *Immun. Ageing* **2021**, *18*, 1. [CrossRef]
23. Trump, S.; Lukassen, S.; Anker, M.S.; Chua, R.L.; Liebig, J.; Thürmann, L.; Corman, V.M.; Binder, M.; Loske, J.; Klasa, C.; et al. Hypertension delays viral clearance and exacerbates airway hyperinflammation in patients with COVID-19. *Nat. Biotechnol.* **2020**. [CrossRef]
24. Zheng, Y.Y.; Ma, Y.T.; Zhang, J.Y.; Xie, X. COVID-19 and the cardiovascular system. *Nat. Rev. Cardiol.* **2020**, *17*, 259–260. [CrossRef] [PubMed]

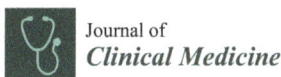

Article

Obesity Strongly Predicts COVID-19-Related Major Clinical Adverse Events in Coptic Clergy

Michael Y. Henein [1,2,3,*], Ibadete Bytyçi [1], Rachel Nicoll [1], Rafik Shenouda [1,4], Sherif Ayad [5], Federico Vancheri [6] and Matteo Cameli [7]

1. Institute of Public Health and Clinical Medicine, Umea University, 90187 Umea, Sweden; i.bytyci@hotmail.com (I.B.); rachelnicoll25@gmail.com (R.N.); rafik.shenouda@umu.se (R.S.)
2. Molecular and Clinic Research Institute, St George University, London SW17 0QT, UK
3. Institute of Fluid Dynamics, Brunel University, London UB8 3PH, UK
4. International Cardiac Centre, Alexandria 21526, Egypt
5. Department of Cardiology, Faculty of Medicine, Alexandria University, Alexandria 21526, Egypt; sherifwagdyayad@yahoo.com
6. Department of Internal Medicine, S. Elia Hospital, 93100 Caltanissetta, Italy; federico.vancheri@ki.se
7. Department of Medical Biotecnologies, Division of Cardiology, University of Siena, 53100 Siena, Italy; matteo.cameli@yahoo.com
* Correspondence: michael.henein@umu.se; Tel.: +46-90-785-14-31

Citation: Henein, M.Y.; Bytyçi, I.; Nicoll, R.; Shenouda, R.; Ayad, S.; Vancheri, F.; Cameli, M. Obesity Strongly Predicts COVID-19-Related Major Clinical Adverse Events in Coptic Clergy. *J. Clin. Med.* **2021**, *10*, 2752. https://doi.org/10.3390/jcm10132752

Academic Editor: Dagmar L. Keller

Received: 29 April 2021
Accepted: 18 June 2021
Published: 22 June 2021

Publisher's Note: MDPI stays neutral with regard to jurisdictional claims in published maps and institutional affiliations.

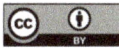

Copyright: © 2021 by the authors. Licensee MDPI, Basel, Switzerland. This article is an open access article distributed under the terms and conditions of the Creative Commons Attribution (CC BY) license (https://creativecommons.org/licenses/by/4.0/).

Abstract: Background and Aims: The Coptic clergy, due to their specific work involving interaction with many people, could be subjected to increased risk of infection from COVID-19. The aim of this study, a sub-study of the COVID-19-CVD international study of the impact of the pandemic on the cardiovascular system, was to assess the prevalence of COVID-19 among Coptic priests and to identify predictors of clinical adverse events. Methods: Participants were geographically divided into three groups: Group-I: Europe and USA, Group II: Northern Egypt, and Group III: Southern Egypt. Participants' demographic indices, cardiovascular risk factors, possible source of infection, number of liturgies, infection management, and major adverse events (MAEs), comprising death, or mechanical ventilation, were assessed. Results: Out of the 1570 clergy serving in 25 dioceses, 255 (16.2%) were infected. Their mean age was 49.5 ± 12 years and mean weekly number of liturgies was 3.44 ± 1.0. The overall prevalence rate was 16.2% and did not differ between Egypt as a whole and overseas ($p = 0.23$). Disease prevalence was higher in Northern Egypt clergy compared with Europe and USA combined (18.4% vs. 12.1%, $p = 0.03$) and tended to be higher than in Southern Egypt (18.4% vs. 13.6%, $p = 0.09$). Ten priests (3.92%) died of COVID-19-related complications, and 26 (10.2) suffered a MAE. The clergy from Southern Egypt were more obese, but the remaining risk factors were less prevalent compared with those in Europe and USA ($p = 0.01$). In multivariate analysis, obesity (OR = 4.180; 2.479 to 12.15; $p = 0.01$), age (OR = 1.055; 0.024 to 1.141; $p = 0.02$), and systemic hypertension (OR = 1.931; 1.169 to 2.004; $p = 0.007$) predicted MAEs. Obesity was the most powerful independent predictor of MAE in Southern Egypt and systemic hypertension in Northern Egypt ($p < 0.05$ for both). Conclusion: Obesity is very prevalent among Coptic clergy and seems to be the most powerful independent predictor of major COVID-19-related adverse events. Coptic clergy should be encouraged to follow the WHO recommendations for cardiovascular disease and COVID-19 prevention.

Keywords: COVID-19; Coptic clergy; prevalence; major adverse events; obesity

1. Introduction

COVID-19 is an aggressive pandemic that has claimed the life of millions worldwide [1]. Virus mutations, a known phenomenon, have now been detected in Europe, Africa, and America, carrying with it doubt about the protective effect of the recently developed vaccines [2,3]. According to the World Health Organization (WHO) recommendations, optimum personal hygiene and physical distancing are the two most important means of preventing virus transmission; hence, the internationally implemented strict lockdowns represent a life-saving strategy despite their drastic impact on the world's economy [4,5].

Coptic priesthood is considered a life vocation with no retirement and with a heavy burden of service involving liturgies, church meetings, home visits, etc. [6]. Furthermore, the nature of the liturgical services requires close contact in the form of touching hands, kissing crosses and icons, and sharing sacramental vessels, a practice that subjects the Coptic clergy to potential infection risk [7,8].

The aim of this study was to assess the prevalence of Coptic clergy who caught COVID-19, irrespective of the clinical management regimen required, home treatment, or hospital admission, to identify the potential risk factors that contributed to disease spread, and to propose practical means for optimum disease prevention.

2. Methods

This is a sub-study within the COVID-19-CVD international study, which investigates the impact of the pandemic on the cardiovascular system, and which has been approved by the Swedish Ethics Board (Dnr 2020-02217 Stockholm avdelning 2 medicin) and the International Cardiac Centre-ICC Ethics Board (ICC, 3/2021, Egypt). M.Y.H. (The Principal Investigator-PI) designed the study protocol, which was endorsed by the Head of the Coptic Church in Egypt. The anonymized data were sent to I.B., a Ph.D. candidate, for statistical analysis.

Since weather conditions and individual habits differ between various regions of Egypt, with some humid (North) and others hot and dry (South), the potential impact of geographic distribution on the prevalence of infection in Egypt and abroad (Europe and the USA) was also assessed (Figure 1). Dioceses in Egypt were divided into two main regions, North, including Alexandria, Delta, and Cairo; and South, including all cities geographically south of Cairo. Data collected from European countries and the USA were presented and analyzed, having been combined together in one group since they mostly followed similar disease prevention and treatment methods, including social distancing. We did not have data on uninfected and asymptomatic but spreadable clergy to compare with infected clergy. The study duration was from March till December 2020.

2.1. Clinical Events

Clinical events (CE) were retrospectively collected while compiling data from dioceses. Information on participants' clinical outcomes were obtained from the medical records, clinical visits, personal communication with general physicians, and telephone interviews with patients and relatives, in a strict confidential way. The primary study end-point was major adverse events (MAEs), defined as the combination of death related to COVID-19 and mechanical ventilation. The secondary clinical outcomes were death, mechanical ventilation, or re-infection.

2.2. Cardiovascular Risk Factors Assessment

Participants' conventional cardiovascular risk factors were assessed as follows: overweight was determined as body mass index (BMI) of 25–29.9 kg/m^2, and obesity was taken as BMI $\geq$ 30 kg/m^2. Systemic hypertension (AH) was diagnosed when systolic blood pressure (SBP) was $\geq$130 mmHg and/or diastolic blood pressure (DBP) was $\geq$80 mmHg or when antihypertensive therapy was prescribed. Diabetes mellitus (DM) was considered based on pre-recruitment diagnosis leading to participants who commenced conventional oral hypoglycemics and/or insulin therapy. Hypercholesterolemia was determined from medical records or if he had been prescribed statins. Evidence for coronary artery disease was also gathered from medical records, based on prior investigations and management.

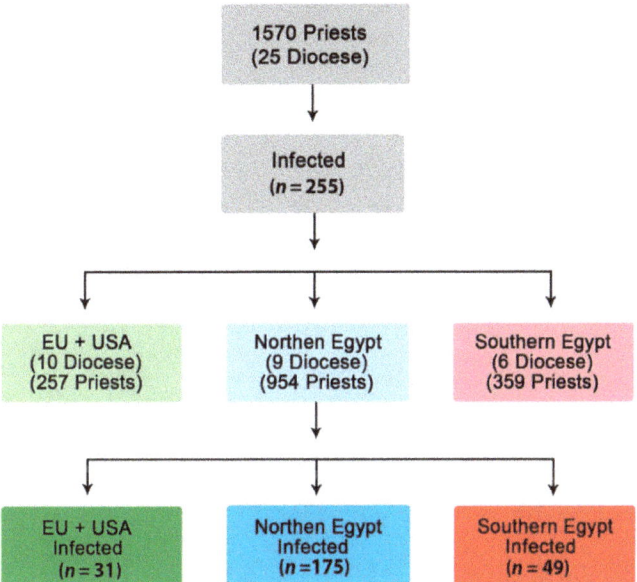

Figure 1. Flow chart of participants.

2.3. Statistical Analysis

Data are summarized using frequencies (percentages) for categorical variables and mean ± standard deviation (SD) for continuous variables or median interquartile (IRQ) ranges. Continuous data were compared with two-tailed Student *t* test and discrete data with chi-square test. Analysis of variance and Bonferroni statistical tests were used to compare quantitative variables between more than two groups. The degree of association between clinical variables and disease prevalence was determined using the Pearson's correlation coefficient in the case of continuous variables; chi-square test (categorical and categorical variables) and point biserial correlation were used in the case of categorical and continuous variables. Predictors of clinical complications (mechanical ventilation) and death were identified with univariate analysis. Independent predictors were identified using multivariate logistic regression analysis using the stepwise method. A significant difference was defined as *p* value < 0.05 (2-tailed). Statistical analysis was performed with SPSS Software Package version 26.0 (IBM Corp., Armonk, NY, USA).

3. Results

3.1. Demographic Indices of the Participating Clergy

Twenty-five dioceses provided data on their affected clergy: 15 from Egypt and 10 from overseas (Europe and USA). Out of the 1570 clergy with available data, 255 (16.2%) were infected with the following likely source of infection: church (30.1%), home (12.8%), and personal contact (16.3%), while the remaining (40.1%) were unknown. The mean age of infected clergy was 49.5 ± 12 years, and the mean weekly number of served liturgies was 3.44 ± 1.0. Two hundred and ten (82.7%) of the infected clergy were treated at home, and the remaining forty-four (17.3%) required hospital admission and management; sixteen (6.72%) of them needed mechanical ventilation. Ten clergy (3.92%) died of COVID-19-related complications, and twenty-six (10.2%) of the infected clergy suffered major adverse events (Table 1).

Table 1. Demographic, clinical, and outcome data of Coptic clergy.

Variable	Priests (n = 255)
Demographic and clinical data	
Age (years)	49.5 ± 12
BMI (m/kg^2)	32 ± 6.2
SBP (mmHg)	127 ± 13
DBP (mmHg)	83 ± 9.5
Underweight (n, %)	0 (0)
Normal weight (n, %)	21 (8.4)
Overweight (n, %)	101 (39.8)
Obese (n, %)	133 (52.2)
AH (n, %)	71 (27.9)
DM (n, %)	60 (23.5)
DM type 1 (n, %)	6 (2.65%)
Dyslipidemia	67 (26.5)
CHD (n, %)	24 (9.6)
Family history for CHD (n, %)	22 (8.9)
Family history for stroke (n, %)	14 (5.8)
Liturgies per week	3.44 ± 1.0
Source of infection	
Home (n, %)	32 (12.8)
Church (n, %)	76 (30.1)
Personal (n, %)	41 (16.3)
Unknown (n, %)	102 (40.1)
Outcome data	
Home treatment (n, %)	210 (82.7)
Hospital treatment (n, %)	44 (17.3)
Intensive care (n, %)	21 (8.4)
Home treatment (days)	17.9 ± 10.3
Hospital treatment (days)	10.2 ± 9.4
Intensive care (days)	7.4 ± 3.4
Mechanical ventilator (n, %)	16 (6.72)
Death (n, %)	10 (3.92)
MAE (n, %)	26 (10.2)

AH: arterial hypertension; BMI: body mass index; CHD; coronary heart disease; DM: diabetes mellitus; SBP: systolic blood pressure; DBP: diastolic blood pressure.

3.2. Impact of Cardiovascular Risk Factors on Disease Prevalence

One hundred and one (39.8%) clergy were overweight, and one hundred and thirty-three (52.2%) were obese. Seventy-one (27.9%) clergy were on anti-hypertensive medications, sixty (23.5%) were treated for diabetes, sixty-seven (26.5%) were treated for dyslipidemia, and twenty-four (9.6%) had a history of coronary artery disease (Table 1). Hypertension measurements, taken at the time of data collection, correlated strongly with the prevalence of COVID-19, SBP (r = 0.78, $p < 0.001$), and DBP (r = 0.74, $p < 0.01$, Figure 2). Similarly, obesity strongly correlated with disease prevalence (r_{pb} = 0.61, p = 0.002, Figure 3). No relationship was found between age, BMI, diabetes, or number of weekly served liturgies and the prevalence of COVID-19 ($p > 0.05$ for all, Table 2). We also tested the possible impact of dioceses with higher disease prevalence on the correlation analysis. In influence analysis, the relationship between diocese prevalence and SBP, DBP, age, and number of liturgies per week showed almost similar correlation, with only small reduction of magnitude with SBP and DBP (Supplementary Materials Figure S1).

3.3. Geographical Impact on Disease Prevalence

The overall prevalence of COVID-19 infection among clergy did not differ between Egypt, as a whole and abroad (p = 0.23). The Northern Egypt clergy had significantly higher disease prevalence compared with the regions of Europe and USA combined (18.4% vs. 12.1%, p = 0.03) and tended to be higher compared with Southern Egypt

(18.4% vs. 13.6%, $p = 0.09$). There was no difference in disease prevalence between Southern Egypt and Europe and USA combined ($p = 0.46$, Figure 4).

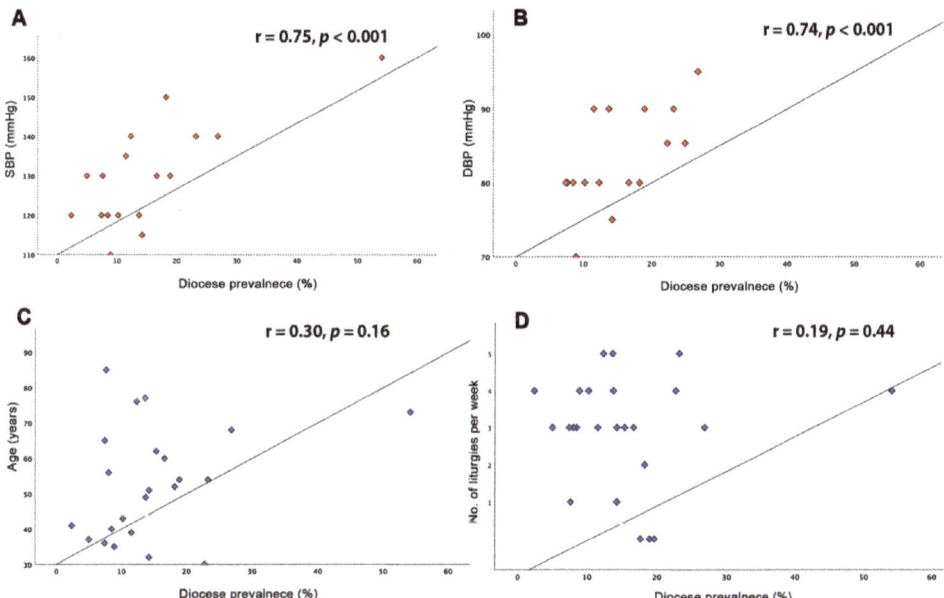

Figure 2. Relationship between risk factors and prevalence of COVID-19 among Clergy. (**A**) Disease prevalence with SBP; (**B**) disease prevalence with DBP; (**C**) disease prevalence with age; (**D**) disease prevalence with number of liturgies per week. SBP: systolic blood pressure; DBP: diastolic blood pressure.

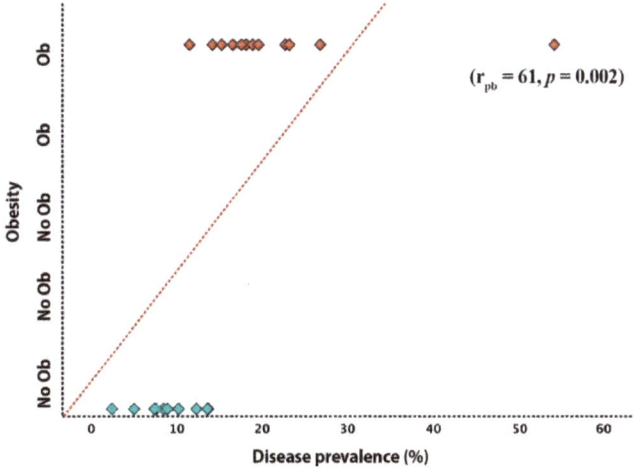

No Ob: no obese; Ob: obese

Figure 3. Relationship between obesity and prevalence of COVID-19 among Clergy.

Table 2. Relationship between prevalence with demographic and clinical variables.

Variable	r	p Value
Age	0.30	0.16
BMI	−0.12	0.57
CHD	−0.38	0.09
DM	0.10	0.68
SBP	0.75	<0.001
DBP	0.74	<0.001
Obesity	0.61	0.002
Liturgies per week	0.19	0.44

BMI: body mass index; CHD: coronary heart disease; DM: diabetes mellitus; SBP: systolic blood pressure; DBP: diastolic blood pressure.

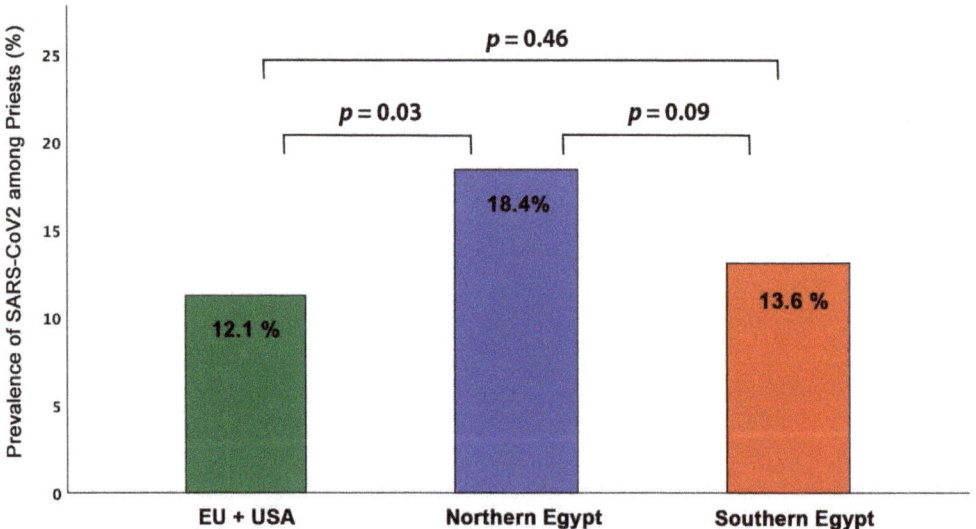

Figure 4. Prevalence of COVID-19 among Clergy in different regions.

We also tested the impact of any dioceses with higher disease prevalence on the overall prevalence of the region. Five of the twenty-five dioceses had high prevalence (above 18%, Supplementary Materials Figure S2): two from Northern Egypt, two from Southern Egypt, and one from the Europe and USA combined group, compared with the remaining dioceses. Obesity tended to be more prevalent ($p = 0.052$) in those five dioceses combined, but the rest of the CV risk factors and demographic indices were not significantly different compared with the rest of the dioceses ($p > 0.05$ for all). Testing the influence analysis, the overall mean between regions proved insignificant (10.8%, 12.9%, 9.2%, respectively, $p > 0.05$ for all), suggesting no significant individual diocesan influence.

In subgroup analysis based on the region where clergy lived and served, no difference was found by subject age, BMI, systolic or diastolic blood pressure, and number of weekly served liturgies ($p > 0.05$ for all) between regions. The clergy from Southern Egypt were more obese compared with those in Europe and USA ($p = 0.01$), but other risk factors were less prevalent compared with Northern Egypt and compared with the combination of Europe and the USA: hypertension (24.3%, 38%, and 36.4%; $p < 0.05$, respectively) and coronary heart disease (2.8%, 11.3%, 9.5%; $p < 0.05$, respectively). The prevalence of diabetes and dyslipidemia was not different between groups according to location (Table 3).

Table 3. Demographic, clinical and outcome data of priests in different regions.

Variable	EU+ USA (n = 31)	Northern Egypt (n = 175)	Southern Egypt (n = 49)	p-Value
Demographic and clinical data				
Age (years)	52.7 ± 11	49.6 ± 12	47.4 ± 11	NS
BMI (m/kg^2)	31 ± 9.1	32 ± 5.7	33 ± 5.3	NS
SBP (mmHg)	126 ± 10	127 ± 14	125 ± 11	NS
DBP (mmHg)	82 ± 6.1	83 ± 9.6	84 ± 11	NS
Underweight (n, %)	0 (0)	0 (0)	0 (0)	NS
Normal weight (n, %)	5 (15.4)	10 (6.10) [a]	5 (11.5)	0.03
Overweight (n, %)	16 (51.6)	72 (41.2) [a]	12 (25.5) [b,c]	0.04
Obese (n, %)	10 (30.7)	92 (52.6) [a]	29 (59.5) [b]	0.02
AH (n, %)	11 (36.4)	66 (38)	12 (24.3) [b,c]	0.001
DM (n, %)	9 (28.6)	46 (26.6)	14 (29.7)	NS
Dyslipidemia	9 (31.8)	60 (34.6) [a]	10 (22.2) [c]	0.03
CHD (n, %)	3 (9.5)	20 (11.36)	1 (2.85) [b,c]	0.004
Family history of CHD (n, %)	7 (23.8)	19 (10.8)	0 (0) [b,c]	0.01
Family history of stroke (n, %)	3 (10.7)	10 (5.92)	9 (4.4) [b]	0.04
Liturgies per week (n, %)	3.6 ± 1.2	3.4 ± 1.0 [a]	3.5 ± 0.8	NS
Source of infection				
Home (n, %)	3 (9.7)	20 (11.7)	13 (28.2) [b,c]	0.02
Church (n, %)	11 (35.5)	54 (30.9)	15 (32.6)	NS
Personal (n, %)	5 (16.1)	32 (18.4)	7 (15.2)	NS
Unknown (n, %)	12 (40.1)	68 (38.9)	11 (23.9) [b,c]	0.001
Outcome data				
Home treatment (n, %)	27 (88)	129 (74.2)	46 (97.7) [c]	0.04
Hospital treatment (n, %)	10 (31.8)	26 (15.1) [a]	8 (18.4)	0.03
Intensive care (n, %)	3 (8.7)	19 (10.8)	5 (10.2)	NS
Home treatment (days)	17.2 ± 11	18.1 ± 11	17.7 ± 6.9	NS
Hospital treatment (days)	12.5 ± 12	9.7 ± 6.4 [a]	8.6 ± 4.5	0.001
Intensive care (days)	4.2 ± 3.9	6.9 ± 3.2	13 ± 8.4 [a]	0.01
Mechanical ventilator (n, %)	2 (4.8)	10 (5.71)	4 (8.2)	NS
Death (n, %)	0 (0)	7 (4.1) [a]	3 (6.4) [b]	<0.001
MAE (n, %)	2 (6.4)	17 (10.2) [a]	7 (14.9) [b,c]	<0.001

[a] $p < 0.05$; Gr. I vs. II, [b] $p < 0.05$; Gr. I vs. III, [c] $p < 0.05$; Gr. II vs. III. AH: arterial hypertension; BMI: body mass index; CHD: coronary heart disease; DM: diabetes mellitus; SBP: systolic blood pressure; DBP: diastolic blood pressure; NS: non significant.

3.4. Predictors of Clinical Events

The overall mortality rate in the study participants was 4.42%, with no difference between Northern and Southern Egypt (4.1% vs. 6.4%, $p > 0.05$) and with 0% mortality in Europe and USA. Likewise, the rate of MAE was 2 times higher in the two Egyptian regions compared with Europe and the USA (12.6% vs. 6.4%, $p < 0.001$). MAEs were significantly higher in Southern Egypt clergy compared with the Northern Egypt clergy (14.9% vs. 10.2%, $p < 0.05$ Table 3).

In univariate analysis, age ($p = 0.003$), CHD ($p = 0.002$), hospital treatment ($p = 0.001$), and mean number of days of home treatment ($p = 0.001$) predicted mortality. In a multivariate analysis model, only hospital treatment (OR 3.116; 2.586 to 4.796; $p = 0.007$) predicted COVID-19 disease-related mortality (Table 4). Age ($p = 0.02$), obesity ($p = 0.02$), CHD ($p = 0.03$), mean days of home treatments ($p = 0.04$), and arterial hypertension ($p = 0.01$) were all predictors of combined MAEs (death and mechanical ventilation), but in multivariate analysis, the independent predictors of MAE were: obesity (OR = 4.180; 2.479 to 12.15; $p = 0.01$), age (OR = 1.055; 0.024 to 1.141; $p = 0.01$), and arterial hypertension (OR = 1.931; 1.169 to 2.004; $p = 0.007$). Testing the impact of geographical distribution on the predictors of COVID-19-related MAE showed that obesity was the most powerful independent predictor in Southern Egypt, and systemic hypertension was the most powerful independent predictor in Northern Egypt. Because of the limited data available, we could not test the

MAE in regions of Europe and USA (Table 5). Collinearity between these measurements was not met based on VIF < 10 for all predictors.

Table 4. Predictors of death among infected clergy.

Variable	Univariate Predictors OR (95% CI)	p-Value	Multivariate Predictors OR (95% CI)	p-Value
Age	1.085 (1.029 to 1.153)	0.003	1.001 (0.918 to 1.092)	0.98
BMI	1.022 (0.925 to 1.130)	0.66		
Diabetes	0.745 (0.045 to 3.706)	0.71		
Obesity	5.461 (1.015 to 16.94)	0.06		
AH	0.511 (0.103 to 2.530)	0.41		
Dyslipidemia	1.070 (0.257 to 4.014)	0.81		
CHD	1.429 (1.271 to 3.144)	0.002	3.007 (0.282 to 6.059)	0.36
No. of liturgies	0.800 (0.415 to 1.541)	0.51		
Home treatment	1.910 (0.232 to 15.74)	0.54		
Hospital treatment	4.615 (3.836 to 5.958)	0.001	3.116 (2.586 to 4.796)	0.007
Mean home days	0.784 (0.671 to 0.915)	0.002	0.922 (0.803 to 1.059)	0.25
Mean hospital days	1.010 (0.928 to 1.100)	0.21		

AH: arterial hypertension; BMI: body mass index; CHD: coronary heart disease; DM: diabetes mellitus; SBP: systolic blood pressure; DBP: diastolic blood pressure.

Table 5. Predictors of MAE among infected clergy.

Variable	Univariate Predictors OR (95% CI)	p-Value	Multivariate Predictors OR (95% CI)	p-Value
Age	1.031 (0.991 to 1.008)	0.04	1.055 (0.024 to 1.141)	0.01
AH	1.938 (1.172 to 2.001)	0.01	1.931 (1.169 to 2.004)	0.007
Diabetes	0.702 (0.222 to 2.170)	0.52		
BMI	1.011 (0.901 to 1.209)	0.26		
Obesity	3.366 (1.055 to 9.785)	0.02	4.180 (2.479 to 12.15)	0.01
Dyslipidemia	0.710 (0.312 to 2.231)	0.55		
CHD	4.122 (1.202 to 15.01)	0.02	3.625 (0.802 to 17.89)	0.09
No. of liturgies	0.608 (0.451 to 1.342)	0.31		
Home days	0.997 (0.806 to 1.011)	0.04	1.480 (0.209 to 7.032)	0.62
Hospital days	0.990 (0.801 to 1.068)	0.33		
Northern Egypt				
Age	1.081 (1.033 to 1.166)	0.003	1.077 (0.980 to 1.613)	0.21
AH	1.520 (1.111 to 2.509)	0.04	1.542 (1.042 to 2.931)	0.03
CHD	1.429 (1.271 to 3.144)	0.002	3.001 (0.200 to 6.012)	0.24
Southern Egypt				
Age	1.011 (0.909 to 1.380)	0.04	2.110 (0.991 to 3.101)	0.31
AH	0.902 (0.400 to 1.970)	0.03	0.809 (0.106 to 2.121)	0.08
Obesity	1.901 (1.001 to 3.122)	0.01	2.990 (1.202 to 3.015)	0.02

MAE: major adverse events (death, re-infection, mechanical ventilation). Not enough data concerning clinical outcome in Europe and USA.

3.5. Comparison with Data from other Communities

Churches around the world had serious loss of life as a result of the pandemic [9], but available official data are very limited. Our results show that the overall prevalence of COVID-19 among Coptic clergy was 14.2% (18.4%, 13.4%, 12.1% for Northern Egypt, Southern Egypt, and combined Europe and USA, respectively). This prevalence is significantly higher than that reported in the UK (7%, $p < 0.001$). Compared with other communities with somewhat shared traditions, Coptic Egypt demonstrated less disease prevalence in the Coptic clergy compared with ultra-Orthodox Jews (constituting 10–12% of inhabitants of Israel) in whom the disease prevalence proved to be 40% [10]. Even in the UK, the disease prevalence rate among ultra-Orthodox Jews in London was reported to be significantly high, approaching 64%, compared with the overall country prevalence of 7% ($p < 0.001$) [11]. Similar comparisons apply to the overall COVID-19-related mortality rate of Italian Catholic clergy, which proved to be significantly lower than in our Coptic clergy [12] in Northern and Southern Egypt (0.66% vs. 4.72% vs. 8.1%, respectively, $p < 0.05$).

4. Discussion

Findings: The findings of this paper can be summarized as showing significantly higher prevalence of COVID-19 infection and mortality rate among Coptic clergy compared with other clergy from overseas and compared with other communities, irrespective of their religion and practices. Furthermore, the two most important risk factors that predicted major clinical adverse events were overweight/obesity and hypertension, although these risk factors were less prevalent in clergy serving in Europe and USA, compared with those serving in Egypt.

Data interpretation: Our three important findings are not independent of each other. Obesity is a recognized risk factor for COVID-19 infection and is associated with poor survival, particularly among patients treated in intensive care units and those requiring mechanical ventilation [13,14]. Obesity is known to be associated with a compromised immune system [15], in addition to the significant buildup of internal body fat, which has its mechanical effect in compromising normal physiological respiration including diaphragmatic and lung function [16,17]. Superspreading events (where, typically, 20% of those infected account for 80% of virus transmission) are triggered by increased exhalation of droplets deriving from airway mucosal surfaces during respiration due to degraded airway lining mucous barrier function. A recent study showed that aerosol exhalation increased with severity of COVID-19 infection and higher elevated BMI-years (BMI multiplied by age), with 18% of subjects, who were both older and with higher BMI, accounting for 80% of the total exhaled bioaerosols [18]. These consequences of overweight and obesity explain the high rate of infection and mortality in the studied Coptic clergy. The second most important predictor of infection was hypertension; again, hypertension has long been known for its effect on cardiac structure and function, as well as kidney function, with resulting complications and compromised body immunity [19,20]. On the other hand, diabetes patients, particularly type 1 patients, are prone to worse outcomes when infected with SARS-CoV2, similar to other respiratory viruses, hence indicating an urgent need to mitigate severe acute respiratory syndrome CoV2 infection risk in this group of patients [21–23]. Because of the low prevalence of diabetes in our study population, particularly type 1 diabetes (2.65%), diabetes was not a key risk factor in predicting major adverse events.

Our results show that COVID-19 disease prevalence and related mortality among Coptic clergy are significantly high compared with clergy from other denominations and also compared with other communities, irrespective of similar cultural habits and geographical location. This should be taken seriously on the basis of the other contributing factors. The Coptic clergy lifestyle is significantly different from that of other clergy and ordinary individuals. Their work is commonly in crowded places, churches, and meeting rooms, and they make many home visits. It also involves frequent touching of sacramental vessels, cloths, crosses, icons, etc. According to the WHO recommendations for the pandemic prevention strategy, such an extent of material/object touching is against all health and sanitary advice and could be explained as a potential cause of infection [3,24]. Furthermore, Coptic clergy have the tradition of growing long beards, which can conceivably be seen as a source of continuous infection, being in close proximity to the priest's breath and salivary droplets while talking or giving a sermon. Furthermore, clergymen frequently tough their beards before greeting others. Adding to this, while the WHO recommends frequent thorough hand washing, this cannot be optimally adhered to because of the long hours clergy spend away from home in service to the community. Finally, the social habits and practices are likely to have played a major role, but in the absence of robust evidence for that we felt reluctant to overemphasize it. The latter point is supported by the lower rate of infection and mortality, as well as the lower prevalence of COVID-19 complications in Coptic clergy serving in Europe and USA, where they abide by local rules, as compared to those serving in Egypt.

The findings of the geographical distribution analysis show significantly higher disease prevalence in Northern Egypt compared with Southern Egypt, with obesity as the only independent predictor of MAE in the south and hypertension as the only independent predictor in the north [25,26]. This highlights the importance of local regional community habits and means of undertaking services. Climate may also have a bearing, with the lower prevalence being found in Southern Egypt, where it is hotter, reflecting the findings of other studies. It is well known that high heat reduces the spread of COVID-19 and that the reduction is assisted by high humidity, as reflected in a recent systematic review [27]. High humidity is a factor in determining COVID-19 infectivity, as dry air is known to enable viral transmission and is associated with impaired mucociliary clearance, innate antiviral defense, and tissue repair function. In this instance, the higher heat of Southern Egypt seems to be a greater factor than the higher humidity of the north [28]. In addition, obesity was less prevalent in Coptic clergy serving in Europe and USA, where there was zero COVID-19-related mortality, suggesting better awareness of disease prevention and healthier lifestyle. Finally, the five dioceses identified with very high (18%) prevalence of infection were evenly distributed in the three regions, which strengthens the relevance of lifestyle impact and the customary habits of Coptic clergy having an additional risk for COVID-19 infection and related mortality.

Clinical implications: Obesity is the major risk factor for COVID-19-related major clinical adverse events, including mortality. Significant changes of lifestyle and dietary habits need to be adopted by Coptic clergy in order to maintain general body health and protect them from other related conditions, e.g., hypertension and diabetes. The strong predictive value of obesity for major clinical adverse events highlights its importance, irrespective of the presence of diabetes, the more commonly investigated disease, suggesting the urgent need for their vaccination to guarantee better prevention.

Limitations: This was a retrospective study, so the amount of data available for analysis was limited. We did not have data on uninfected and asymptomatic but spreadable clergy, which would have provided a more accurate and meaningful comparison. Detailed information on clinical care, blood analyses, and accurate assessment of the means of infection were based on the data provided by the clergy themselves rather than using a centralized approach. The small sample size did not allow us to test the impact of geographical distribution among Coptic clergy in Europe and USA. Not all dioceses complied with the request to provide data, so we relied on the available information from 25 dioceses only to run the statistical analyses and document the results for the benefit of Coptic and other clergy. PCR testing was not available in all clergy, but diagnosis and treatment was designed based on clinical findings and antibody detection.

Conclusions: Obesity is very prevalent among Coptic clergy and seems to be the most powerful independent predictor of major COVID-19-related adverse events. Furthermore, because of the nature of their lifestyle, Coptic clergy represent a high-risk group for COVID-19, highlighting the need for stringent management of cardiovascular risk factors according to the well-established WHO recommendations.

Supplementary Materials: The following are available online at https://www.mdpi.com/article/10.3390/jcm10132752/s1, Figure S1: Influence analysis (without dioceses with high prevalence disease) of relationship between risk factors and prevalence of COVID-19 among clergy, Figure S2. Prevalence of SARS-CoV2 among priests in different diocese.

Author Contributions: M.Y.H.: Conceptualization, study design, methodology and project administration; I.B.; R.S., S.A.; data sorting and statistical analysis; I.B., R.N., S.A., F.V.; M.C.; data analysis and writing the first draft of manuscript. All authors contributed to writing and approved the manuscript. All authors have read and agreed to the published version of the manuscript.

Funding: This research received no external funding.

Institutional Review Board Statement: The study was conducted according to the guidelines of the Declaration of Helsinki and approved by the Swedish Ethics Board (Dnr 2020-02217 Stockholm avdelning 2 medicin).

Informed Consent Statement: Informed consent was obtained from all subjects involved in the study.

Data Availability Statement: Not applicable.

Conflicts of Interest: The authors have no conflict of interest to declare.

References

1. Wang, C.; Horby, P.W.; Hayden, F.G.; Gao, G.F. A novel coronavirus outbreak of global health concern. *Lancet* **2020**, *395*, 470–473. [CrossRef]
2. Peters, A.; Vetter, P.; Guitart, C.; Lotfinejad, N.; Pittet, D. Understanding the emerging coronavirus: What it means for health security and infection prevention. *J. Hosp. Infect.* **2020**, *104*, 440–448. [CrossRef]
3. Tartari, E.; Muthukumaran, P.; Peters, A.; Allegranzi, B.; Pittet, D. Monitoring your institution: The WHO hand hygiene self-assessment framework—Is it worth it? *Clin. Microbiol. Infect.* **2019**, *25*, 925–928. [CrossRef] [PubMed]
4. WHO. Infection Prevention and Control during Health Care when Novel Coronavirus (Ncov) Infection Is Suspected. Interim Guidance, 2020. Available online: https://apps.who.int/iris/rest/bitstreams/1266296/retrieve (accessed on 25 January 2020).
5. World Health Organization. Coronavirus Disease (COVID-19) Dashboard. Available online: https://covid19.who.int/ (accessed on 9 January 2021).
6. Ratzinger, J.C. *The Spirit of the Liturgy by Joseph Cardinal Ratzinger*; Amazon: Seattle, WA, USA, 2000; p. 174.
7. Aherfi, S.; Gautret, P.; Chaudet, H.; Raoult, D.; La Scola, B. Clusters of COVID-19 associated with Purim celebration in the Jewish community in Marseille, France, March 2020. *Int. J. Infect. Dis.* **2020**, *100*, 88–94. [CrossRef]
8. Budaev, S. Safety and Reverence: How Roman Catholic Liturgy Can Respond to the COVID-19 Pandemic. *J. Relig. Health* **2021**, 1–22. [CrossRef]
9. Biagioni, M.C. 400 Priests Have Died from Covid-19: "Stories of Heroes That Helped Everyone Keep Hope Alive. Available online: https://www.agensir.it/europa/2020/09/29/400-priests-have-died-from-covid-19-stories-of-heroes-that-helped-everyone-keep-hope-alive/ (accessed on 29 September 2020).
10. Rosenberg, D. The Government Can't Save Ultra-Orthodox Jews from COVID-19. Religious Leaders Can. Available online: https://foreignpolicy.com/2020/10/12/the-government-cant-save-ultra-orthodox-jews-from-covid-19-religious-leaders-can/ (accessed on 20 April 2021).
11. Burgess, K. 64% of London's Ultra-Orthodox Jews Infected with Covid. *The Times*. 3 February 2021. Available online: https://www.thetimes.co.uk/article/64-of-londons-ultra-orthodox-jews-infected-with-covid-5dhkw3lz0 (accessed on 20 April 2021).
12. Bramstedt, K.A. COVID-19 as a Cause of Death for Catholic Priests in Italy: An Ethical and Occupational Health Crisis. *Health Soc. Care Chaplain.* **2020**, *8*, 180–190. [CrossRef]
13. Monteiro, A.C.; Suri, R.; Emeruwa, I.O.; Stretch, R.J.; Cortes-Lopez, R.Y.; Sherman, A.; Lindsay, C.C.; Fulcher, J.A.; Goodman-Meza, D.; Sapru, A.; et al. Obesity and smoking as risk factors for invasive mechanical ventilation in COVID-19: A retrospective, observational cohort study. *PLoS ONE* **2020**, *15*, e0238552. [CrossRef]
14. King, C.S.; Sahjwani, D.; Brown, A.W.; Feroz, S.; Cameron, P.; Osborn, E.; Desai, M.; Djurkovic, S.; Kasarabada, A.; Hinerman, R.; et al. Outcomes of mechanically ventilated patients with COVID-19 associated respiratory failure. *PLoS ONE* **2020**, *15*, e0242651. [CrossRef]
15. Stefan, N.; Birkenfeld, A.L.; Schulze, M.B.; Ludwig, D.S. Obesity and impaired metabolic health in patients with COVID-19. *Nat. Rev. Endocrinol.* **2020**, *16*, 341–342. [CrossRef]
16. Simonnet, A.; Chetboun, M.; Poissy, J.; Raverdy, V.; Noulette, J.; Duhamel, A.; Labreuche, J.; Mathieu, D.; Pattou, F.; Jourdain, M.; et al. High Prevalence of Obesity in Severe Acute Respiratory Syndrome Coronavirus-2 (SARS-CoV-2) Requiring Invasive Mechanical Ventilation. *Obesity* **2020**, *28*, 1195–1199. [CrossRef]
17. Belanger, M.J.; Hill, M.A.; Angelidi, A.M.; Dalamaga, M.; Sowers, J.R.; Mantzoros, C.S. Covid-19 and Disparities in Nutrition and Obesity. *N. Engl. J. Med.* **2020**, *383*, e69. [CrossRef] [PubMed]
18. Edwards, D.A.; Ausiello, D.; Salzman, J.; Devlin, T.; Langer, R.; Beddingfield, B.J.; Fears, A.C.; Doyle-Meyers, L.A.; Redmann, R.K.; Killeen, S.Z.; et al. Exhaled aerosol increases with COVID-19 infection, age, and obesity. *Proc. Natl. Acad. Sci. USA* **2021**, *118*, 2021830118. [CrossRef]
19. Schiffrin, E.L.; Flack, J.M.; Ito, S.; Muntner, P.; Webb, R.C. Hypertension and COVID-19. *Am. J. Hypertens.* **2020**, *33*, 373–374. [CrossRef]
20. Kamyshnyi, A.; Krynytska, I.; Matskevych, V.; Marushchak, M.; Lushchak, O. Arterial Hypertension as a Risk Comorbidity Associated with COVID-19 Pathology. *Int. J. Hypertens.* **2020**, *2020*, 8019360. [CrossRef] [PubMed]
21. Drucker, D.J. Diabetes, obesity, metabolism, and SARS-CoV-2 infection: The end of the beginning. *Cell Metab.* **2021**, *33*, 479–498. [CrossRef]
22. Gregory, J.M.; Slaughter, J.C.; Duffus, S.H.; Smith, T.J.; LeStourgeon, L.M.; Jaser, S.S.; McCoy, A.B.; Luther, J.M.; Giovannetti, E.R.; Boeder, S.; et al. COVID-19 Severity Is Tripled in the Diabetes Community: A Prospective Analysis of the Pandemic's Impact in Type 1 and Type 2 Diabetes. *Diabetes Care* **2021**, *44*, 526–532. [CrossRef] [PubMed]

23. Carey, I.M.; Critchley, J.; Dewilde, S.; Harris, T.; Hosking, F.J.; Cook, D.G. Risk of Infection in Type 1 and Type 2 Diabetes Compared with the General Population: A Matched Cohort Study. *Diabetes Care* **2018**, *41*, 513–521. [CrossRef]
24. Islam, M.S.; Rahman, K.M.; Sun, Y.; Qureshi, M.O.; Abdi, I.; Chughtai, A.A.; Seale, H. Current knowledge of COVID-19 and infection prevention and control strategies in healthcare settings: A global analysis. *Infect. Control. Hosp. Epidemiol.* **2020**, *41*, 1196–1206. [CrossRef]
25. Zhao, L.; Stamler, J.; Yan, L.L.; Zhou, B.; Wu, Y.; Liu, K.; Daviglus, M.L.; Dennis, B.H.; Elliott, P.; Ueshima, H.; et al. Blood pressure differences between northern and southern Chinese: Role of dietary factors: The International Study on Macronutrients and Blood Pressure. *Hypertension* **2004**, *43*, 1332–1337. [CrossRef]
26. Elliott, P.; Kesteloot, H.; Appel, L.J.; Dyer, A.R.; Ueshima, H.; Chan, Q.; Brown, I.J.; Zhao, L.; Stamler, J. Dietary phosphorus and blood pressure: International study of macro- and micro-nutrients and blood pressure. *Hypertension* **2008**, *51*, 669–675. [CrossRef]
27. Mecenas, P.; Bastos, R.T.D.R.M.; Vallinoto, A.C.R.; Normando, D. Effects of temperature and humidity on the spread of COVID-19: A systematic review. *PLoS ONE* **2020**, *15*, e0238339. [CrossRef] [PubMed]
28. Chan, K.H.; Peiris, J.S.M.; Lam, S.Y.; Poon, L.L.M.; Yuen, K.Y.; Seto, W.H. The Effects of Temperature and Relative Humidity on the Viability of the SARS Coronavirus. *Adv. Virol.* **2011**, *2011*, 734690. [CrossRef] [PubMed]

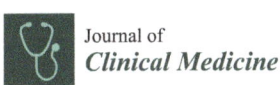

Review

ACE2, the Counter-Regulatory Renin–Angiotensin System Axis and COVID-19 Severity

Filippos Triposkiadis [1,*], Andrew Xanthopoulos [1], Grigorios Giamouzis [1], Konstantinos Dean Boudoulas [2], Randall C. Starling [3], John Skoularigis [1], Harisios Boudoulas [2] and Efstathios Iliodromitis [4]

[1] Department of Cardiology, Larissa University General Hospital, 41110 Larissa, Greece; andrewvxanth@gmail.com (A.X.); grgiamouzis@gmail.com (G.G.); iskoular@gmail.com (J.S.)
[2] Department of Medicine/Cardiovascular Medicine, The Ohio State University, Columbus, OH 43210, USA; Konstantinos.Boudoulas@osumc.edu (K.D.B.); boudoulas@bioacademy.gr (H.B.)
[3] Kaufman Center for Heart Failure Treatment and Recovery, Heart, Vascular, and Thoracic Institute, Cleveland Clinic, Cleveland, OH 44195, USA; starlir@ccf.org
[4] Second Department of Cardiology, National and Kapodistrian University of Athens, Attikon University Hospital, 12462 Athens, Greece; iliodromitis@yahoo.gr
* Correspondence: ftriposkiadis@gmail.com

Abstract: Angiotensin (ANG)-converting enzyme (ACE2) is an entry receptor of severe acute respiratory syndrome coronavirus 2 (SARS-CoV-2) that causes coronavirus disease 2019 (COVID-19). ACE2 also contributes to a deviation of the lung renin–angiotensin system (RAS) towards its counter-regulatory axis, thus transforming harmful ANG II to protective ANG (1–7). Based on this purported ACE2 double function, it has been put forward that the benefit from ACE2 upregulation with renin–angiotensin–aldosterone system inhibitors (RAASi) counterbalances COVID-19 risks due to counter-regulatory RAS axis amplification. In this manuscript we discuss the relationship between ACE2 expression and function in the lungs and other organs and COVID-19 severity. Recent data suggested that the involvement of ACE2 in the lung counter-regulatory RAS axis is limited. In this setting, an augmentation of ACE2 expression and/or a dissociation of ACE2 from the ANG (1–7)/Mas pathways that leaves unopposed the ACE2 function, the SARS-CoV-2 entry receptor, predisposes to more severe disease and it appears to often occur in the relevant risk factors. Further, the effect of RAASi on ACE2 expression and on COVID-19 severity and the overall clinical implications are discussed.

Keywords: COVID-19; ACE2; renin–angiotensin system

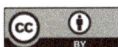

1. Introduction

The rapid spread of severe acute respiratory syndrome coronavirus 2 (SARS-CoV-2) has led to a sudden outbreak of coronavirus disease 2019 (COVID-19) that has affected the entire world. COVID-19 clinical manifestations range from asymptomatic infection to severe disease, with pneumonia and acute respiratory distress syndrome (ARDS) set in motion by inflammation, large-vessel thrombosis, and in situ microthrombi [1].

SARS-CoV-2, which is usually transmitted by respiratory particles released from an infected subject, initially targets the nasal multiciliated epithelial cells [2]. Subsequently, the infection spreads to the upper airways and in selected patients to the deepest parts of the lungs, where it targets the type II pneumocytes causing severe pneumonia and acute respiratory distress syndrome (ARDS) [3]. Finally, massive systemic multiorgan infection may occur, as the virus targets the epithelial cells and the endothelial cells of the capillaries [4], the two main components of tissue barriers which are of utmost importance for health [5]. The infection and damage of cells of tissue barriers allow the virus entrance to the bloodstream and lymphatic system, spreading to several organs including the heart [6], the kidney [7], and the brain [8,9]. This mechanism may also explain why pulmonary infection can occur after functional exclusion of the upper airways from the lungs (e.g., after total laryngectomy) [10]. It should be noted, however, that viremia is not the main route of SARS-CoV-2 spreading [11].

The SARS-CoV-2 enters the host cells through binding to the angiotensin-converting enzyme (ACE2) receptor after activation of the S1 domain of SARS-CoV-2 spike (S) protein by an ACE2 co-factor, the transmembrane protease serine 2 (TMPRSS2) [12,13]. The ACE2 receptor, however, is an important member of the counter-regulatory axis of the renin–angiotensin system (RAS), which parallel to its pivotal function in fluid volume control, plays a major role for other functions as well, including stem cell maintenance and differentiation, hematopoiesis, vasculogenesis, erythropoiesis, myeloid differentiation, inflammation, and innate and adaptive immunity, among others [14,15].

It has been posited that down-regulation of membrane-bound ACE2 by SARS-CoV-2 eliminates the function of the counter-regulatory RAS axis, that in turn escalates the severity of the inflammation observed in SARS-CoV-2 [16,17]. It has been suggested that the renin–angiotensin–aldosterone system (RAAS) inhibitors (RAASi), including ACE inhibitors (ACEi), angiotensin II (ANG II) receptor blockers (ARB), and mineralocorticoid receptor antagonists (MRA), increase ACE2 receptor expression [18–20], and thus, the benefits from the anti-inflammatory effects originating from upregulation of the counter-regulatory RAS axis may counterbalance the risks when using RAASi in the COVID-19 era [21].

In this manuscript we discuss the relationship between ACE2 expression and function in the lungs and other organs and COVID-19 severity. Recent data suggested that the involvement of ACE2 in the lung counter-regulatory RAS axis is limited. In this setting, an augmentation of ACE2 expression and/or a dissociation of ACE2 from the ANG (1–7)/Mas pathways that leaves unopposed the ACE2 function, the SARS-CoV-2 entry receptor, predisposes to more severe disease and it appears to often occur in the relevant risk factors. Further, the effect of RAASi on ACE2 expression and on COVID-19 severity and the overall clinical implications are discussed.

2. The Lung Counter-Regulatory RAS AXIS and COVID-19

According to the classic view, RAS is a sequence of assorted enzymatic steps that build up in the production of a single biologically active metabolite, the octapeptide angiotensin ANG II, by ACE [22]. However, new roles for certain intermediate products have been disclosed [23]; they may be processed in different ways by various enzymes, the most well-known being the ACE homolog ACE2. One effect is to set up a second counter-regulatory axis through ACE2/ANG (1–7), whose end-point metabolite ANG (1–7) occupies MAS receptors. ACE2 and other enzymes can generate ANG (1–7) directly or indirectly from either the decapeptide ANG I or from ANG II that acts on the receptor MAS to regulate multiple mechanisms in the heart, kidney, brain, and other tissues. In many cases, this counter-regulatory axis appears to compensate for or adjust the effects of the classical axis by mediating protective effects including vasodilation, improvement of endothelial function, inhibition of smooth muscle cell hypertrophy and migration, as well as inhibition of inflammation and thrombosis [23]. However, this may not occur in the lungs, and for this reason an augmentation of membranous ACE2 expression cannot be a therapeutic option, as is discussed in the following sections.

2.1. The SARS-CoV-2 Induced ACE2 Downregulation Is of Doubtful Relevance

It has been surmised that the harmful effects of SARS-CoV-2 are due to ACE2 down-regulation that takes place after virus entrance into the cell by endocytosis [24]. However, various studies employing miscellaneous technologies demonstrated that ACE2 expression in the lungs is low. Hikmet and colleagues assessed the expression pattern of ACE2 covering > 150 different cell types commensurate to all major human tissues and organs [25]. ACE2 expression was for the most part observed in enterocytes, renal tubules, gallbladder, cardiomyocytes, male reproductive cells, placental trophoblasts, ductal cells, eye, and vasculature, whereas in the respiratory system, the ACE2 expression was finite [25]. In another study, the ACE2:ACE ratio in the lungs was 1:20, whereas in kidneys the ACE2:ACE ratio was roughly 1:1 [26]. In the respiratory system, ACE2 protein is abundant within regions of the sinonasal cavity, whereas in the lung parenchyma, ACE2 protein is located in a small subset of alveolar type II cells colocalized with TMPRSS2, a cofactor for SARS-CoV2 entry (Figure 1) [27,28]. Ultimately, ACE2 expression levels are low in the lung AT2, being 4.7-fold lower than the average expression level of all ACE2 expressing cell types [29].

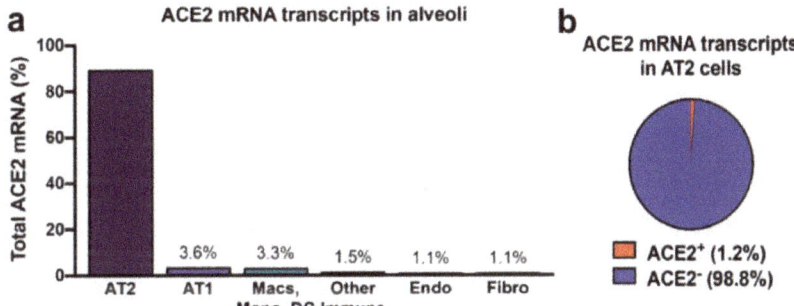

Figure 1. Angiotensin-converting enzyme (ACE)2 expression in human lung. (**a**) Approximately 89.5% of the cells with detectable ACE2 mRNA in the alveoli are alveolar type II cells. (**b**) Only 1–2% of alveolar type II cells have ACE2 mRNA transcripts. Abbreviations: AT2, alveolar type II; AT1, alveolar type I; Macs, Macrophages; Mono, Monocytes; DC, dendritic cells.; Other immune cells, B cells, mast cells, natural killer/T cells; Endo; Endothelial; Fibro, Fibroblasts/myofibroblasts [27].

Considering that SARS-CoV-2 and other viruses that enter via the lung use ACE2 as receptors, the low levels of ACE2 in the lung might help to restrict entry and impart an evolutionary gain in survival. This assumption is further supported by experimental studies demonstrating that lineages of transgenic (Tg) mice expressing high human ACE2 (hACE2; AC70 mice) demonstrated significantly higher lethality post-SARS-CoV infection than the lineages with low hACE2 expression (AC22 mice) [30,31]. Viral replication in the lungs reached a maximum at day 1 post-infection (p.i.), in which averages of $10^{8.5}$ and $10^{8.7}$ tissue culture infective doses (TCID$_{50}$) SARS-CoV/gram were recovered from AC70 and AC22 mice, respectively, and gradually declined thereafter. However, at day 5 p.i. a significantly higher level of viral replication was sustained in the lungs of a single AC70 mouse than any AC22 mice [31].

2.2. The Binding of SARS-CoV-2 with ACE2 May Ignite a Catastrophic Inflammatory Response

SARS-CoV-2 induced cell destruction triggers a local immune response characterized by recruitment of macrophages and monocytes that release cytokines and prime adaptive T and B cell immune responses contributing in most cases to the final elimination of the pathogen [32,33]. However, in certain instances, especially if risk factors (e.g, old age, smoking, pollutants, other) are involved, there is inefficacious control of viral replication, viral propagation and eventually infection of the lower airways. Viral escape is accompanied by a huge release of pro-inflammatory cytokines (sepsis-like inflammation or cytokine storm) due to hyperactivation of the innate immune system and along with the inhibition of the adaptive immune response may result in severe disease and/or death [34].

In autopsy of patients who succumbed to severe acute respiratory syndrome, SARS-CoV S protein and its RNA were only detected in ACE2$^+$ cells in the lungs and other organs, and high levels of proinflammatory cytokines were exclusively detected in the SARS-CoV-infected ACE2$^+$ cells [35]. Expression of ACE2 is tightly linked to innate and acquired immune responses, regulation of B cell-mediated immunity, and cytokine secretion, indicating that an elevated expression of ACE2 may lengthen the virus life cycle, intensify virus replication, and bring about entry of the virus into the host cell [36,37]. Taken together, occupation of ACE2 by SARS-Cov-2 may ignite inflammatory signaling, and any intervention elevating lung ACE2 expression may amplify this process.

2.3. Prolyloligopeptidase (POP), Also Named Prolylendopeptidase, Rather Than ACE2 Seems to Underlie ANG (1–7) Generation in the Lungs

A recent ex vivo study examined the partial contribution to ANG (1–7) generation from ANG II by ACE2 and POP in serum, kidney, and lung tissues. POP, and not ACE2, was the principal enzyme responsible for ANG II transformation to ANG (1–7) in the circulation and the lungs [38]. In the same study, it was also demonstrated that POP is significantly less effective in transforming the harmful ANG II to the protective ANG (1–7) compared with ACE2.

POP is a cytoplasmic enzyme, but its activity can also be quantified in body fluids. Peptides up to 30 amino acids long that contain a proline are potential substrates of POP. Many years of experimental work have indicated that POP has not a single physiologically distinguishing role but several roles depending on the milieu in which POP is located [39]. Moreover, POP is proinflammatory as it concurrently participates in the generation of the matrikine proline-glycine-proline (PGP) from collagen fragments; (PGP) has traditionally been characterized as a neutrophil chemoattractant [40]. The commencing cleavage of native collagen by matrix metalloproteinases (MMPs) originates from a variety of cellular elements producing appropriately sized substrate fragments for POP that subsequently act to free PGP followed by acetylation and transformation to acetyl PGP (AcPGP), which is 4–7-fold more potent.

2.4. ACE2 Contributes to SARS-CoV-2 Dissemination within the Organism

Flow cytometry studies have demonstrated marked upregulation of ACE2 expression on the activated alveolar macrophages (significantly higher in the inflammatory M1 than in the anti-inflammatory M2 macrophages), with little to no expression of ACE2 on most of the human peripheral blood-derived immune cells (e.g., CD4+ T, CD8+ T, activated CD4+/CD8+ T, Tregs, Th17, NKT, B, NK cells, monocytes, dendritic cells, and granulocytes) [41]. Accordingly, alveolar macrophages, by virtue of their polarization state toward either an M1 or M2 phenotype, function in a different way following SARS-CoV-2 infection. M1 alveolar macrophages are hijacked by SARS-CoV-2, allowing the viral infection and spread, whereas M2 alveolar macrophages degrade the virus and limit its spread [42]. Thus, while macrophages play an important role in antiviral defense mechanisms, in the case of SARS-CoV-2 due to ACE2 overexpression in the M1 type, they may also serve as a Trojan horse by enabling pulmonary SARS-CoV-2 invasion, facilitating engraftment, producing prolonged local and systemic uncontrolled inflammatory responses, and therefore governing the severity of infection [43].

Thus, from a (patho)physiological point-of-view an increase in the membrane bound ACE2, the SARS-CoV-2 receptor, in the lungs will most likely increase susceptibility to COVID-19 [44], as it is dubious whether it will bolster the counter-regulatory RAS axis (Figure 2) [38,45].

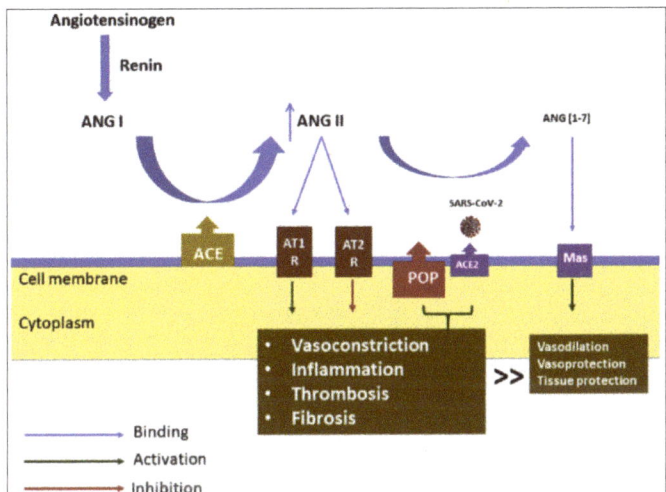

Figure 2. The counter-regulatory renin–angiotensin system (RAS) axis in the lungs in the coronavirus disease 2019 (COVID-19) setting. Angiotensin-converting enzyme 2 (ACE2) serves as the severe acute respiratory syndrome coronavirus (SARS-CoV)-2 receptor, whereas the proinflammatory prolyloligopeptidase (POP) converts less effectively than ACE2 the deleterious angiotensin (ANG) II to the protective ANG (1–7). As a result, deleterious signalling (inflammation, thrombosis and fibrosis) dominates over protective (vasodilation, vasoprotection and tissue protection) signalling in patients with severe COVID-19, which may lead to acute lung injury. Abbreviations: AT1R, angiotensin receptor type 1; AT2R, angiotensin receptor type 2 [45].

3. ACE2 Expression and the Counter-Regulatory RAS AXIS in States Predisposed to Severe COVID-19

There is compelling evidence that cancer, chronic obstructive pulmonary disease (COPD), chronic kidney disease (CKD), heart disease, obesity (body mass index (BMI) ≥ 30 kg/m^2), type 2 diabetes mellitus (T2DM) and solid organ transplantation place adults of any age at increased risk of severe illness from SARS-CoV-2 [46].

3.1. Cancer

In cancer patients with COVID-19, all-cause mortality is high and related to general and cancer-specific risk factors [47]. Some of the general risk factors include age, male sex, number of comorbidities, cardiopulmonary disease, and smoking status, whereas cancer-specific features that have been identified as being associated with worse outcomes include tumour stage, disease progression, and type of cancer; some studies identify thoracic cancers as being associated with increased risk compared with other solid tumors [48].

The RAS is indispensable for stem cell maintenance and differentiation and plays a crucial role in tumorigenesis and cancer progression, suggesting that these roles may intersect and result in regulation of cancer stem cell (CSC) function by the RAS [15]. Elements of the RAS are highly expressed in many cancer types. ACE2 expression is raised in non-small cell lung cancer including adenocarcinoma and squamous cell carcinoma [49]. Moreover, a recent study reported that ACE2 and TMPRSS2 levels are higher at resection margins of lung cancer survivors than those in normal tissues of non-cancerous individuals [50].

Based on comprehensive promoter analysis of ACE-2, Gottschalk and colleagues proposed that STAT3-mediated upregulation of ACE2 might play a critical role both in COVID-19 infection and lung tumor progression [51]. In this regard, SARS-CoV-2 infection might stimulate the binding of STAT3 in the promoter of ACE2, resulting in enhanced expression of ACE-2, which in turns upscales virus entry through the ACE2 receptor. On the other hand, cancer pathologies in lung tissue also switch on the transcription of STAT3, leading to the upregulated expression of ACE2 in cancer cells [51].

ACE2 expression is also raised in renal cancer and gastrointestinal cancer [52]. It is noteworthy that ACE2 and TMPRSS2 are expressed at high levels on tumor and normal colorectal epithelial tissues and that patients with colorectal cancer and COVID-19 are more likely to have lymphopenia, higher respiratory rate, and high hypersensitive C-reactive protein levels than matched patients with COVID-19 but without cancer [53,54]. Finally, landscape profiling analyses on the expression level of ACE2 in pan-cancers have revealed that the risk for development of SARS-CoV-2 infection was coupled with the expression level of ACE2 [36].

3.2. Chronic Obstructive Pulmonary Disease

COPD is a significant risk factor for hospitalization, intensive care unit stay, and mortality in patients with COVID-19 [55,56].

COPD patients are usually cigarette smokers, though long-term exposure to other lung irritants, such as secondhand smoke, is also responsible for COPD development. Pulmonary ACE2 gene expression is upregulated in ever-smokers compared with non-smokers irrespective of COPD status [57]. A meta-analysis demonstrated a 25% increase in pulmonary ACE2 expression in ever-smokers and a trend for higher ACE2 levels in COPD patients [57]. In another study ACE2 mRNA expression was significantly higher in the lung tissue of current smokers without airflow limitation and current smokers with COPD (GOLD stages II and III–IV) as compared with never-smokers. In addition, ex-smokers without airflow limitation had significantly lower ACE2 mRNA levels as compared with current smokers [58]. Leung and colleagues investigated gene expression levels of ACE-2 in the airways of individuals with and without COPD in three different cohorts and found that COPD and current smokers had significantly increased expression of ACE-2 [59]. Importantly, gene expression levels of ACE-2 were inversely related to an individual's forced expiratory volume 1 (FEV1), suggesting a dose-dependent response. Lastly, a differential expression of ACE2 and TMPRSS2 in nasal and bronchial airways relative to age and disease status was reported. Children were found to have significantly lower expression of COVID-19 receptors in the upper and lower airways (nasal and bronchial). Moreover, the lung airway expression of both ACE2 and TMPRSS2 was found to be significantly upregulated in smokers compared with non-smokers, and in patients with COPD compared with healthy subjects [60]. Likewise, Fliesser and colleagues observed increased ACE2 and TMPRSS2 expression in lung tissue with a concomitant decrease in protective sACE2 in COPD patients [61].

3.3. Chronic Kidney Disease

CKD has come up not only as the most prevalent comorbidity carrying an increased risk for severe COVID-19, but also as the comorbidity that imparts the highest risk of severe COVID-19 [62].

ACE2 is predominantly expressed in the brush border of proximal tubular cells, less in the podocytes and vascular endothelial cells, and not at all in the glomerular endothelial and mesangial cells [63]. The functional role of ACE2 in the kidney has not been delineated. Although ACE2 has been described as a crucial player in the enzymatic conversion of ANG II to ANG (1–7), this may not be the case in the kidney, in which neprilysin (NEP) seems to be the major source of renal ANG (1–7) [64]. Indeed, it is estimated that in the healthy human kidneys, ACE2, prolylcarboxypeptidase (PCP), and POP together contribute less than 15% of total ANG (1–7) production [65].

There is severe RAS dysregulation in CKD [65]. In normal subjects, overall kidney ANG (1–7) generation exceeds ANG II generation by 2.6-fold and is 3.9 times higher than in CKD, indicating preponderance of the counter-regulatory RAS axis in healthy kidneys (Figure 3). In contrast, in CKD patients, chymase-dependent ANG II generation is 4.5 times higher than generation by ACE, which is compatible with serious RAS dysregulation.

POP-mediated ANG (1–7) generation is extremely low. ACE2 and PCP-mediated ANG II to ANG (1–7) transformation is present at a higher level in CKD than in healthy kidneys, albeit minor compared with NEP activity. Collectively these findings suggest that both in normal subjects and patients with CKD the contribution of ACE2 to the renal counter-regulatory ANG (1–7)/Mas axis is limited.

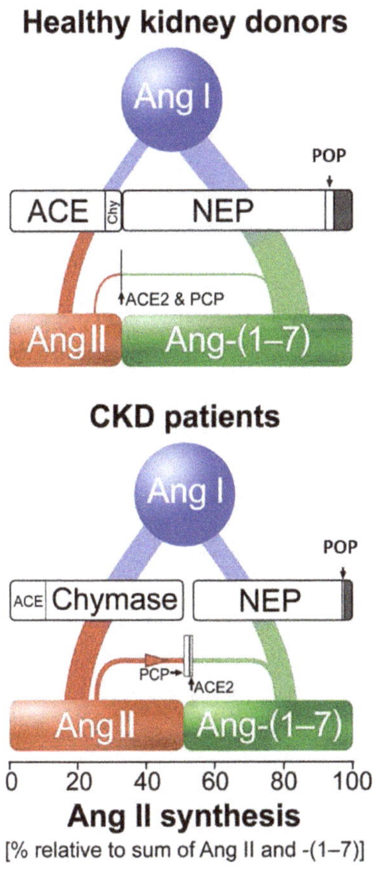

Figure 3. Overview of angiotensin processing by kidney-resident enzymes. Comparison of relative Ang (angiotensin) II and Ang (1–7) synthesis from Ang I in healthy kidney donors (top) and patients with chronic kidney disease (CKD; bottom). In healthy kidney donors, Ang I is mainly converted by NEP (neprilysin) to Ang (1–7) and to a smaller degree by ACE (angiotensin-converting enzyme) to Ang II. Minor contribution by chymase and POP (prolyl-endopeptidase) supplement Ang II and (1–7) synthesis, respectively. ACE2 and PCP (prolyl-carboxypeptidase)-mediated Ang II to Ang (1–7) conversion is present at a very low degree. Overall, the pathways producing Ang (1–7) exceed those which produce Ang II. B, In patients with CKD, Ang I is equally converted by chymase to Ang II and by NEP to Ang (1–7). Ang II synthesis is dominated by chymase and supplemented by ACE. POP-mediated Ang (1–7) synthesis is present at a very low degree. ACE2 and PCP-mediated Ang II to Ang (1–7) conversion is present at a higher degree than in healthy kidneys, albeit still minor in comparison to neprilysin's activity. Thus, in comparison to healthy kidney donors, in patients with CKD severe renin–angiotensin system (RAS) dysregulation is exhibited, characterized by low Ang (1–7) production and high chymase-mediated Ang II production. In both cohorts, one or more unidentified enzymes contribute to a small portion of Ang I to Ang (1–7) conversion (depicted by gray area). The horizontal dimensions of the boxes equal median enzyme contribution [65].

Tissue expression of ACE2 and TMPRSS2 were analyzed in renal tubulointerstitial and glomerular microarray expression data of healthy living donors (HLD) and patients with CKD obtained from the European Renal cDNA Bank. ACE2 expression was similar in the tubulointerstitium of the two groups, but lower in glomeruli of CKD patients compared to HLD. TMPRSS2 expression was similar in the tubulointerstitium but lower in glomeruli of CKD patients compared to HLD and there was a strong relationship between ACE2 and TMPRSS2 expression in the glomerulus [66]. Based on these findings it has been conjectured that the colocalization and co-expression of ACE2 and TMPRSS2 in the glomerulus and their strong correlation in this compartment may underlie the recent clinical observation of an emerging SARS-CoV-2-associated nephropathy (COVAN) [67].

3.4. Cardiac Disease

Many patients with COVID-19 suffer from underlying cardiac disease or develop acute cardiac injury during the course of the illness [68].

Cardiac ACE2 expression is highest in pericytes, but also detectable in vascular smooth muscle cells, fibroblasts, and cardiomyocytes [69]. In an experimental model of heart failure (HF), ACE2 immunoreactivity and mRNA levels increased in pulmonary, cardiac, and renal tissues in compensated but not in decompensated HF [70]. Elevated cardiac ACE2 expression at both mRNA and protein levels has also been reported in human HF [71]. Examination of the distribution of the cardiac ACE2 expression levels in dilated cardiomyopathy and hypertrophic cardiomyopathy has affirmed downregulation of ACE2 expression in fibroblasts, pericytes, and vascular smooth muscles with a concomitant upregulation of ACE2 expression in cardiomyocytes [72]. Similar findings have been reported in patients with aortic stenosis and HF with reduced ejection fraction [73].

A recent experimental study investigated the expression of several enzymes including ACE2 and TMPRSS2 in the lung, heart and kidneys of male Sprague Dawley rats with chronic HF created by a surgical aorto-caval fistula. Sham-operated rats served as controls [70]. ACE2 immunoreactivity and mRNA levels increased in pulmonary, cardiac and renal tissues of compensated but not of decompensated chronic HF. Interestingly, both the expression and abundance of pulmonary, cardiac and renal TMPRSS2 decreased in chronic HF in correlation with the severity of the disease. The authors conjectured that the increased expression of the ACE2 together with the suppression of TMPRSS2, which facilitates SARS-CoV-2 entry into ACE2, in HF may serve as a compensatory mechanism, counterbalancing the over-activity of the deleterious isoform, ACE [70].

3.5. Obesity

Obese individuals with COVID-19 are more likely to require hospital admission and intensive care unit stay and have increased mortality compared with healthy weight individuals [74].

Obesity is associated with an imbalance of the RAAS system [75]. Moreover, a recent experimental study found that the ACE2 expression was significantly higher in obese male mice relative to lean male controls or to obese female mice, whereas expression of TMPRSS2 in trachea was significantly lower in obese male mice relative to lean male controls and obese female mice. The authors proposed that these observations may potentially account, at least in part, for the association of obesity with SARS-CoV-2 infection and COVID-19 severity, as well as the male-biased mortality rate and that other cellular proteases may potentially contribute to SARS-CoV-2 entry into the TMPRSS2-negative cells [76].

ACE2 is broadly expressed in the adipose tissue and significantly more in the visceral than peripheral subcutaneous adipose tissue [77]. Consequently, obese individuals, especially those with visceral obesity, can acquire more viral load, which probably contributes to the increased COVID-19 severity compared with normal weight individuals [78]. Importantly, RAAS system imbalance reverses after weight loss [79].

3.6. Type 2 Diabetes Mellitus

T2DM is associated with poor outcomes after COVID-19 infection and with an increase in time required for viral clearance. T2DM is linked to raised ACE2 expression [80].

Experimental studies demonstrated that mice with diabetes have upregulated ACE2 and TMPRSS2 both in the lungs and the kidney [81]. In lung tissue samples, pulmonary ACE2 mRNA expression was similar between individuals with and without diabetes, whereas protein levels of ACE2 were significantly higher in both alveolar tissue and bronchial epithelium in individuals with diabetes; these findings were independent of smoking, COPD, BMI, RAASi use, and other potential confounders [82].

3.7. Solid Organ Transplantation

During the COVID-19 pandemic, concerns about adverse outcomes among organ transplant recipients, difficulties with infection prevention and control, and decreased resource availability led to a profound reduction in deceased donor organ transplantation, which was associated with a rise in waitlist deaths [83]. However, transplantation has currently returned to pre-2020 levels, reflecting the increasing understanding of the transplant community of the risks of deferring transplantation for patients on waiting lists [84].

Local RAS regulation is profoundly modified in solid organ transplant recipients. Heart transplant recipients are at a higher risk of SARS-COV-2 infection and have a twofold higher mortality in comparison to the general population if they acquire the disease [85]. Early after kidney transplantation (KTx), ANG II generation within the graft is ACE-mediated, while ANG (1–7) generation is dominantly mediated by NEP from ANG II. In aged allografts, a strong increase in local chymase-mediated ANG II synthesis associated with constant high NEP-mediated ANG (1–7) synthesis occurs [86]. Chymase expression may not only enhance local ANG II formation, but also restrict NEP/ANG (1–7)-mediated alternative RAS activation by exhausting ANG I as a substrate for NEP. Post-cardiac transplantation (HTx) patients with acute rejection show increased ACE activity but not ACE2, whereas those with chronic allograft vasculopathy show increased ACE2 activity [87].

However, despite the previously mentioned derangements, there is currently limited evidence supporting an independent relationship between the timing of transplant or recent induction immunosuppression and mortality from COVID-19. In general, the preponderance of evidence supports that age and coexisting morbidities, rather than immunosuppression, drive COVID-19 mortality among solid organ transplant recipients [84].

4. ACE2 and RAAS Inhibitors

Some early experimental studies demonstrated elevated expression of ACE2, the SARS-CoV-2 receptor, following the use of RAASi, raising concerns regarding the safety of these agents that currently form the backbone for the treatment of hypertension and HF in the COVID-19 era [18,20]. Current evidence regarding the potential of these agents to facilitate disease contraction and modify disease severity has been based on observational studies with the well-known significant limitations and on small, randomized control trials.

The RAASi controversy during the COVID-19 outbreak was most likely unjustifiable after all, as recent data suggest that these drugs do not increase ACE2 expression. In the kidney cortex of mice receiving captopril or telmisartan there was no increase in ACE2 activity and protein compared with control mice [88]. In healthy young mice, neither the ACEi ramipril nor the ARB telmisartan affected lung or kidney ACE2 or TMPRSS2, except for a small increase in kidney ACE2 protein with ramipril [81]. In contrast, mice with comorbid diabetes had heightened lung ACE2 and TMPRSS2 protein levels and increased lung ACE2 activity. None of these parameters were affected by RAS blockade. ACE2 was similarly upregulated in the kidneys of mice with comorbid diabetes compared with aged controls, whereas TMPRSS2 (primarily distal nephron) was highest in telmisartan-treated animals [81].

Examination of ACE2 gene expression in lung tissue samples revealed that ACEi and ARB did not enhance ACE2 expression (Figure 4) [89]. Likewise, there was no association between renal expression of ACE2 and either hypertension or common types of RAASi in kidney transcriptomes [90]; in another study, ACE2 expression was unaffected by either ACEi or ARB therapy [91]. In nasal cavity tissues and in the paranasal sinuses obtained both from healthy control donors and patients with chronic rhinosinusitis, the use of ACEi or ARB did not increase the expression of ciliary ACE2 receptors [92]. Finally, ACEi may increase ANG (1–7), the effector peptide product of ACE2, by inhibiting its degradation by ACE into angiotensin [1–5,93]. Regarding spironolactone, there is evidence to suggest that it may be protective in the COVID-19 setting by downregulating the androgen promoter of TMPRSS2 by its antiandrogenic actions and upregulating protease nexin 1 or serpin E2 (PN1), which in turn inhibits furin and plasmin, two of the processors of the spike protein [94]. Collectively, the above studies strongly support the notion that RAASi do not increase ACE2 expression and that the initial concerns regarding this issue were exaggerated.

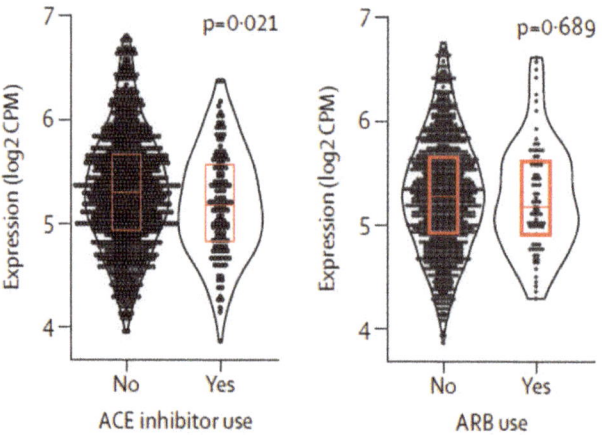

Figure 4. Effects of ACE inhibitor use, and ARB use on the expression of SARS-CoV-2 receptor (ACE2) in human lung tissue. Superimposed box plots show median (IQR). p values are from robust linear models, adjusted for current smoking status. ACE inhibitor use was associated with significantly lower ACE2 expression, whereas ARB was not. Abbreviations: ACE, angiotensin-converting enzyme; ARB, angiotensin II receptor blocker; CPM, counts per million; SARS-CoV-2, severe acute respiratory syndrome coronavirus 2 [89].

5. Clinical Implications

SARS-CoV-2 entry into ACE2, which is upregulated in many risk factors predisposing to severe COVID-19, is facilitated by TMPRSS2-induced activation of the S protein via its serine protease activity. This traditional observation suggests that the modulation of TMPRSS2 expression may furnish an alternative strategy to treat SARS-CoV-2 infection by blocking viral entry into host cells (Figure 5) [95]. The initial experimental data suggest that this treatment approach may be promising.

The hepatocyte growth factor activator inhibitor 2 (HAI-2) is a cognate inhibitor of TM-PRSS2 [96]. In an experimental study expression of HAI-2 in human lung adenocarcinoma Calu-3 cells was knocked down (KD) by small interfering RNA transfection, and SARS-CoV-2 infection assays were performed. The level of viral RNA in HAI-2 KD cells was approximately 40 times greater than that in control cells, indicating that the endogenous level of HAI-2 in Calu-3 cells alleviated SARS-CoV-2 infection [97]. In accordance with the previous findings, some small molecules (e.g., homoharringtonine and halofuginone) that reduce surface expression of TMPRSS2 render cells exposed to them at drug concentrations known to be achievable in human plasma markedly resistant to SARS-CoV-2 infection in both live and pseudoviral in vitro models [98].

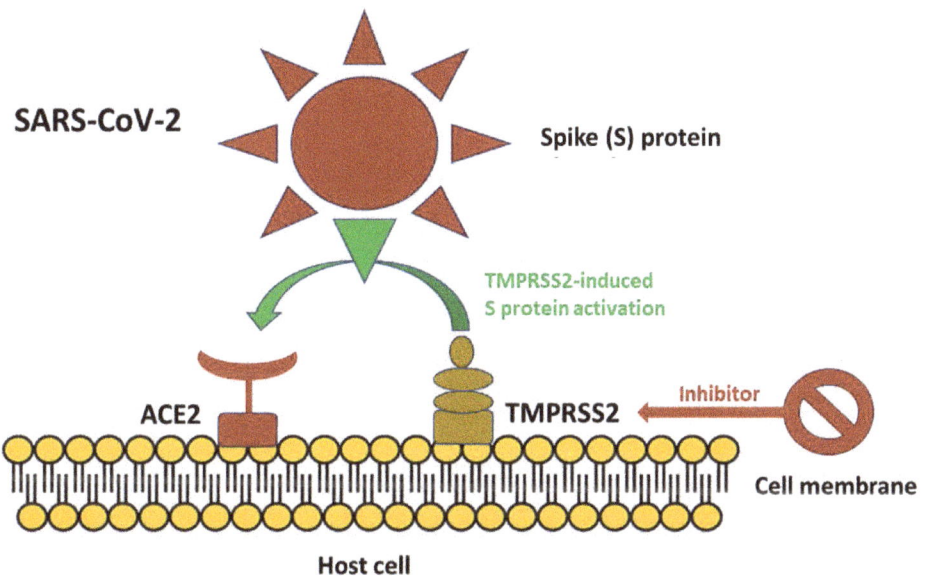

Figure 5. SARS-CoV-2 entry into ACE2 is facilitated by TMPRSS2 induced activation of the S protein via its serine protease activity. Inhibition of TMPRSS2 may furnish an alternative strategy to treat SARS-CoV-2 infection by blocking viral entry into host cells.

Based on the encouraging preliminary results, in a recent study a comprehensive structural modeling and binding-site analysis of the serine protease TMPRSS2 was performed, followed by a structure-based virtual screening against the National Center for Advancing Translational Sciences (NCATS) library consisting of up to 200,000 drug-like compounds designed from a diverse chemical space [99]. Selected hits were evaluated in the TMPRSS2 biochemical assay and the SARS-CoV-2-S pseudotyped particle entry assay, and a number of novel inhibitors were identified, providing a starting point for the further development of therapeutic drug candidates for COVID-19.

6. Conclusions

The SARS-CoV-2 enters ACE2, the main SARS-CoV-2 receptor, following primings of the viral S protein by the ACE2 cofactor TMPRSS2. ACE2 is additionally a crucial enzymatic player in several organs moving the RAS towards the counter-regulatory RAS axis by enzymatically transforming ANG II to ANG (1–7). However, this may not be the case in the lungs and kidneys, organs whose function is a major determinant of COVID-19 severity and outcome, where it predominantly serves as the SARS-CoV-2 receptor (Figure 6). Medical conditions and disease states associated with severe COVID-19 are characterized by an increase in ACE2 expression, dissociation of ACE2 from the ANG (1–7)/Mas pathway, or both. RAASi do not appear to affect COVID-19 severity by affecting lung ACE2 expression. The encouraging experimental results with agents that target TMPRSS2 should help expedite the rational design of human clinical trials designed to combat SARS-CoV-2 entry into ACE2 and active COVID-19 infection.

❖ ACE2 is a SARS-CoV-2 receptor.

❖ ACE2 in the lungs is expressed in a small subset of ATII cells (arrow).

❖ It is doubtful whether ACE2 contributes to conversion of ANGII to ANG (1-7) in the lungs.

❖ An increase in lung ACE2 solely increases SARS-CoV-2 receptor abundance. RAASi do not increase lung ACE2.

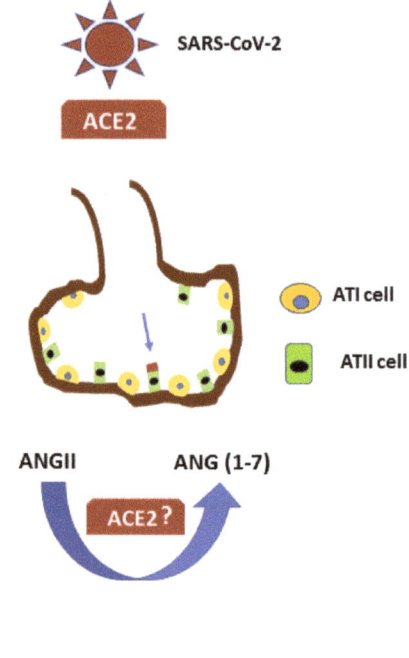

Figure 6. Expression and function of ACE2 in the lungs in the coronavirus disease 2019 (COVID-19) era. Abbreviations: ACE2, angiotensin-converting enzyme 2; SARS-CoV-2, severe acute respiratory distress syndrome coronary virus 2; ATI cell, lung alveolar epithelial type I cell; ATII cell, lung alveolar epithelial type II cell; ANG, angiotensin; RAASi, renin–angiotensin–aldosterone system inhibitors.

Funding: This research received no external funding.

Institutional Review Board Statement: Not applicable.

Informed Consent Statement: Not applicable.

Conflicts of Interest: The authors declare no conflict of interest.

Abbreviations

ACE: angiotensin-converting enzyme; ACEi: ACE inhibitors; AcPGP: acetyl PGP; ANG II: angiotensin II; ARB: angiotensin II receptor blockers; ARDS: acute respiratory distress syndrome; CKD: chronic kidney disease; COPD: chronic obstructive pulmonary disease; COVID-19: coronavirus disease 2019; ICU: intensive care unit; MMPs: matrix metalloproteinases; MRA: mineralocorticoid receptor antagonists; POP: Prolyloligopeptidase; RAS: renin–angiotensin system; RAASi: renin–angiotensin–aldosterone system inhibitors; SARS-CoV-2: severe acute respiratory syndrome coronavirus 2; STAT3: Signal Transducer And Activator Of Transcription 3; T2DM: type 2 diabetes mellitus; TMPRSS2: transmembrane protease serine 2.

References

1. Connors, J.M.; Levy, J.H. COVID-19 and its implications for thrombosis and anticoagulation. *Blood* **2020**, *135*, 2033–2040. [CrossRef]
2. Ahn, J.H.; Kim, J.; Hong, S.P.; Choi, S.Y.; Yang, M.J.; Ju, Y.S.; Kim, Y.T.; Kim, H.M.; Rahman, M.D.T.; Chung, M.K.; et al. Nasal ciliated cells are primary targets for SARS-CoV-2 replication in the early stage of COVID-19. *J. Clin. Investig.* **2021**, *131*. [CrossRef]
3. Marcinkiewicz, J.; Witkowski, J.M.; Olszanecki, R. The dual role of the immune system in the course of COVID-19. The fatal impact of the aging immune system. *Cent. Eur. J. Immunol.* **2021**, *46*, 1–9. [CrossRef] [PubMed]
4. Chilosi, M.; Poletti, V.; Ravaglia, C.; Rossi, G.; Dubini, A.; Piciucchi, S.; Pedica, F.; Bronte, V.; Pizzolo, G.; Martignoni, G.; et al. The pathogenic role of epithelial and endothelial cells in early-phase COVID-19 pneumonia: Victims and partners in crime. *Mod. Pathol.* **2021**, *34*, 1444–1455. [CrossRef] [PubMed]
5. Garcia-Ponce, A.; Chanez Paredes, S.; Castro Ochoa, K.F.; Schnoor, M. Regulation of endothelial and epithelial barrier functions by peptide hormones of the adrenomedullin family. *Tissue Barriers* **2016**, *4*, e1228439. [CrossRef] [PubMed]
6. Lindner, D.; Fitzek, A.; Brauninger, H.; Aleshcheva, G.; Edler, C.; Meissner, K.; Scherschel, K.; Kirchhof, P.; Escher, F.; Schultheiss, H.P.; et al. Association of Cardiac Infection With SARS-CoV-2 in Confirmed COVID-19 Autopsy Cases. *JAMA Cardiol.* **2020**, *5*, 1281–1285. [CrossRef]
7. Diao, B.; Wang, C.; Wang, R.; Feng, Z.; Zhang, J.; Yang, H.; Tan, Y.; Wang, H.; Wang, C.; Liu, L.; et al. Human kidney is a target for novel severe acute respiratory syndrome coronavirus 2 infection. *Nat. Commun.* **2021**, *12*, 2506. [CrossRef]
8. Erickson, M.A.; Rhea, E.M.; Knopp, R.C.; Banks, W.A. Interactions of SARS-CoV-2 with the Blood-Brain Barrier. *Int. J. Mol. Sci.* **2021**, *22*, 2681. [CrossRef]
9. Reza-Zaldivar, E.E.; Hernandez-Sapiens, M.A.; Minjarez, B.; Gomez-Pinedo, U.; Marquez-Aguirre, A.L.; Mateos-Diaz, J.C.; Matias-Guiu, J.; Canales-Aguirre, A.A. Infection Mechanism of SARS-COV-2 and Its Implication on the Nervous System. *Front. Immunol.* **2020**, *11*, 621735. [CrossRef] [PubMed]
10. Gallo, O.; Trotta, M.; Orlando, P.; Maggiore, G.; Bicci, E.; Locatello, L.G. SARS-CoV-2 in upper and lower airway samples of a laryngectomized patient: New insights and many lessons. *Oral Oncol.* **2020**, *107*, 104841. [CrossRef] [PubMed]
11. Bermejo-Martin, J.F.; Gonzalez-Rivera, M.; Almansa, R.; Micheloud, D.; Tedim, A.P.; Dominguez-Gil, M.; Resino, S.; Martin-Fernandez, M.; Ryan Murua, P.; Perez-Garcia, F.; et al. Viral RNA load in plasma is associated with critical illness and a dysregulated host response in COVID-19. *Crit. Care* **2020**, *24*, 691. [CrossRef]
12. Li, W.; Moore, M.J.; Vasilieva, N.; Sui, J.; Wong, S.K.; Berne, M.A.; Somasundaran, M.; Sullivan, J.L.; Luzuriaga, K.; Greenough, T.C.; et al. Angiotensin-converting enzyme 2 is a functional receptor for the SARS coronavirus. *Nature* **2003**, *426*, 450–454. [CrossRef]
13. Matsuyama, S.; Nao, N.; Shirato, K.; Kawase, M.; Saito, S.; Takayama, I.; Nagata, N.; Sekizuka, T.; Katoh, H.; Kato, F.; et al. Enhanced isolation of SARS-CoV-2 by TMPRSS2-expressing cells. *Proc. Natl. Acad. Sci. USA* **2020**, *117*, 7001–7003. [CrossRef] [PubMed]
14. Bernstein, K.E.; Khan, Z.; Giani, J.F.; Cao, D.Y.; Bernstein, E.A.; Shen, X.Z. Angiotensin-converting enzyme in innate and adaptive immunity. *Nat. Rev. Nephrol.* **2018**, *14*, 325–336. [CrossRef] [PubMed]
15. Roth, I.M.; Wickremesekera, A.C.; Wickremesekera, S.K.; Davis, P.F.; Tan, S.T. Therapeutic Targeting of Cancer Stem Cells via Modulation of the Renin-Angiotensin System. *Front. Oncol.* **2019**, *9*, 745. [CrossRef]
16. Zipeto, D.; Palmeira, J.D.F.; Arganaraz, G.A.; Arganaraz, E.R. ACE2/ADAM17/TMPRSS2 Interplay May Be the Main Risk Factor for COVID-19. *Front. Immunol.* **2020**, *11*, 576745. [CrossRef] [PubMed]
17. Yan, T.; Xiao, R.; Lin, G. Angiotensin-converting enzyme 2 in severe acute respiratory syndrome coronavirus and SARS-CoV-2: A double-edged sword? *FASEB J.* **2020**, *34*, 6017–6026. [CrossRef] [PubMed]
18. Ferrario, C.M.; Jessup, J.; Chappell, M.C.; Averill, D.B.; Brosnihan, K.B.; Tallant, E.A.; Diz, D.I.; Gallagher, P.E. Effect of angiotensin-converting enzyme inhibition and angiotensin II receptor blockers on cardiac angiotensin-converting enzyme 2. *Circulation* **2005**, *111*, 2605–2610. [CrossRef]
19. Ferrario, C.M.; Jessup, J.; Gallagher, P.E.; Averill, D.B.; Brosnihan, K.B.; Ann Tallant, E.; Smith, R.D.; Chappell, M.C. Effects of renin-angiotensin system blockade on renal angiotensin-(1-7) forming enzymes and receptors. *Kidney Int.* **2005**, *68*, 2189–2196. [CrossRef]
20. Keidar, S.; Gamliel-Lazarovich, A.; Kaplan, M.; Pavlotzky, E.; Hamoud, S.; Hayek, T.; Karry, R.; Abassi, Z. Mineralocorticoid receptor blocker increases angiotensin-converting enzyme 2 activity in congestive heart failure patients. *Circ. Res.* **2005**, *97*, 946–953. [CrossRef] [PubMed]
21. Brojakowska, A.; Narula, J.; Shimony, R.; Bander, J. Clinical Implications of SARS-CoV-2 Interaction With Renin Angiotensin System: JACC Review Topic of the Week. *J. Am. Coll. Cardiol.* **2020**, *75*, 3085–3095. [CrossRef] [PubMed]
22. Chappell, M.C. Nonclassical renin-angiotensin system and renal function. *Compr. Physiol.* **2012**, *2*, 2733–2752. [CrossRef]
23. Santos, R.A.S.; Sampaio, W.O.; Alzamora, A.C.; Motta-Santos, D.; Alenina, N.; Bader, M.; Campagnole-Santos, M.J. The ACE2/Angiotensin-(1-7)/MAS Axis of the Renin-Angiotensin System: Focus on Angiotensin-(1-7). *Physiol. Rev.* **2018**, *98*, 505–553. [CrossRef] [PubMed]
24. Chaudhry, F.; Lavandero, S.; Xie, X.; Sabharwal, B.; Zheng, Y.Y.; Correa, A.; Narula, J.; Levy, P. Manipulation of ACE2 expression in COVID-19. *Open Heart* **2020**, *7*. [CrossRef]

25. Hikmet, F.; Mear, L.; Edvinsson, A.; Micke, P.; Uhlen, M.; Lindskog, C. The protein expression profile of ACE2 in human tissues. *Mol. Syst. Biol.* **2020**, *16*, e9610. [CrossRef]
26. Malha, L.; Mueller, F.B.; Pecker, M.S.; Mann, S.J.; August, P.; Feig, P.U. COVID-19 and the Renin-Angiotensin System. *Kidney Int. Rep.* **2020**, *5*, 563–565. [CrossRef] [PubMed]
27. Ortiz, M.E.; Thurman, A.; Pezzulo, A.A.; Leidinger, M.R.; Klesney-Tait, J.A.; Karp, P.H.; Tan, P.; Wohlford-Lenane, C.; McCray, P.B., Jr.; Meyerholz, D.K. Heterogeneous expression of the SARS-Coronavirus-2 receptor ACE2 in the human respiratory tract. *EBioMedicine* **2020**, *60*, 102976. [CrossRef]
28. Zhao, Y.; Zhao, Z.; Wang, Y.; Zhou, Y.; Ma, Y.; Zuo, W. Single-Cell RNA Expression Profiling of ACE2, the Receptor of SARS-CoV-2. *Am. J. Respir. Crit. Care Med.* **2020**, *202*, 756–759. [CrossRef]
29. Qi, F.; Qian, S.; Zhang, S.; Zhang, Z. Single cell RNA sequencing of 13 human tissues identify cell types and receptors of human coronaviruses. *Biochem. Biophys. Res. Commun.* **2020**, *526*, 135–140. [CrossRef]
30. Tseng, C.T.; Huang, C.; Newman, P.; Wang, N.; Narayanan, K.; Watts, D.M.; Makino, S.; Packard, M.M.; Zaki, S.R.; Chan, T.S.; et al. Severe acute respiratory syndrome coronavirus infection of mice transgenic for the human Angiotensin-converting enzyme 2 virus receptor. *J. Virol.* **2007**, *81*, 1162–1173. [CrossRef]
31. Yoshikawa, N.; Yoshikawa, T.; Hill, T.; Huang, C.; Watts, D.M.; Makino, S.; Milligan, G.; Chan, T.; Peters, C.J.; Tseng, C.T. Differential virological and immunological outcome of severe acute respiratory syndrome coronavirus infection in susceptible and resistant transgenic mice expressing human angiotensin-converting enzyme 2. *J. Virol.* **2009**, *83*, 5451–5465. [CrossRef] [PubMed]
32. Gallo, O.; Locatello, L.G.; Mazzoni, A.; Novelli, L.; Annunziato, F. The central role of the nasal microenvironment in the transmission, modulation, and clinical progression of SARS-CoV-2 infection. *Mucosal Immunol.* **2021**, *14*, 305–316. [CrossRef]
33. Tay, M.Z.; Poh, C.M.; Renia, L.; MacAry, P.A.; Ng, L.F.P. The trinity of COVID-19: Immunity, inflammation and intervention. *Nat. Rev. Immunol.* **2020**, *20*, 363–374. [CrossRef] [PubMed]
34. Manjili, R.H.; Zarei, M.; Habibi, M.; Manjili, M.H. COVID-19 as an Acute Inflammatory Disease. *J. Immunol.* **2020**, *205*, 12–19. [CrossRef]
35. He, L.; Ding, Y.; Zhang, Q.; Che, X.; He, Y.; Shen, H.; Wang, H.; Li, Z.; Zhao, L.; Geng, J.; et al. Expression of elevated levels of pro-inflammatory cytokines in SARS-CoV-infected ACE2+ cells in SARS patients: Relation to the acute lung injury and pathogenesis of SARS. *J. Pathol.* **2006**, *210*, 288–297. [CrossRef]
36. Dai, Y.J.; Hu, F.; Li, H.; Huang, H.Y.; Wang, D.W.; Liang, Y. A profiling analysis on the receptor ACE2 expression reveals the potential risk of different type of cancers vulnerable to SARS-CoV-2 infection. *Ann. Transl. Med.* **2020**, *8*, 481. [CrossRef]
37. Iwasaki, M.; Saito, J.; Zhao, H.; Sakamoto, A.; Hirota, K.; Ma, D. Inflammation Triggered by SARS-CoV-2 and ACE2 Augment Drives Multiple Organ Failure of Severe COVID-19: Molecular Mechanisms and Implications. *Inflammation* **2021**, *44*, 13–34. [CrossRef]
38. Serfozo, P.; Wysocki, J.; Gulua, G.; Schulze, A.; Ye, M.; Liu, P.; Jin, J.; Bader, M.; Myohanen, T.; Garcia-Horsman, J.A.; et al. Ang II (Angiotensin II) Conversion to Angiotensin-(1-7) in the Circulation Is POP (Prolyloligopeptidase)-Dependent and ACE2 (Angiotensin-Converting Enzyme 2)-Independent. *Hypertension* **2020**, *75*, 173–182. [CrossRef] [PubMed]
39. Garcia-Horsman, J.A. The role of prolyl oligopeptidase, understanding the puzzle. *Ann. Transl. Med.* **2020**, *8*, 983. [CrossRef]
40. O'Reilly, P.J.; Hardison, M.T.; Jackson, P.L.; Xu, X.; Snelgrove, R.J.; Gaggar, A.; Galin, F.S.; Blalock, J.E. Neutrophils contain prolyl endopeptidase and generate the chemotactic peptide, PGP, from collagen. *J. Neuroimmunol.* **2009**, *217*, 51–54. [CrossRef]
41. Song, X.; Hu, W.; Yu, H.; Zhao, L.; Zhao, Y.; Zhao, X.; Xue, H.H.; Zhao, Y. Little to no expression of angiotensin-converting enzyme-2 on most human peripheral blood immune cells but highly expressed on tissue macrophages. *Cytom. A* **2020**. [CrossRef]
42. Lv, J.; Wang, Z.; Qu, Y.; Zhu, H.; Zhu, Q.; Tong, W.; Bao, L.; Lv, Q.; Cong, J.; Li, D.; et al. Distinct uptake, amplification, and release of SARS-CoV-2 by M1 and M2 alveolar macrophages. *Cell Discov.* **2021**, *7*, 24. [CrossRef]
43. Abassi, Z.; Knaney, Y.; Karram, T.; Heyman, S.N. The Lung Macrophage in SARS-CoV-2 Infection: A Friend or a Foe? *Front. Immunol.* **2020**, *11*, 1312. [CrossRef] [PubMed]
44. Beyerstedt, S.; Casaro, E.B.; Rangel, E.B. COVID-19: Angiotensin-converting enzyme 2 (ACE2) expression and tissue susceptibility to SARS-CoV-2 infection. *Eur. J. Clin. Microbiol. Infect. Dis.* **2021**, *40*, 905–919. [CrossRef] [PubMed]
45. Triposkiadis, F.; Starling, R.C.; Xanthopoulos, A.; Butler, J.; Boudoulas, H. The Counter Regulatory Axis of the Lung Renin-Angiotensin System in Severe COVID-19: Physiopathology and Clinical Implications. *Heart Lung Circ.* **2020**. [CrossRef]
46. Pitt, B.; Rossignol, P. Mineralocorticoid Receptor Antagonists in High-Risk Heart Failure Patients With Diabetes Mellitus and/or Chronic Kidney Disease. *J. Am. Heart Assoc.* **2017**, *6*. [CrossRef] [PubMed]
47. Kuderer, N.M.; Choueiri, T.K.; Shah, D.P.; Shyr, Y.; Rubinstein, S.M.; Rivera, D.R.; Shete, S.; Hsu, C.Y.; Desai, A.; de Lima Lopes, G., Jr.; et al. Clinical impact of COVID-19 on patients with cancer (CCC19): A cohort study. *Lancet* **2020**, *395*, 1907–1918. [CrossRef]
48. Lee, A.J.X.; Purshouse, K. COVID-19 and cancer registries: Learning from the first peak of the SARS-CoV-2 pandemic. *Br. J. Cancer* **2021**, *124*, 1777–1784. [CrossRef]
49. Zhang, H.; Quek, K.; Chen, R.; Chen, J.; Chen, B. Expression of the SAR2-Cov-2 receptor ACE2 reveals the susceptibility of COVID-19 in non-small cell lung cancer. *J. Cancer* **2020**, *11*, 5289–5292. [CrossRef] [PubMed]
50. Wang, Q.; Li, L.; Qu, T.; Li, J.; Wu, L.; Li, K.; Wang, Z.; Zhu, M.; Huang, B.; Wu, W.; et al. High Expression of ACE2 and TMPRSS2 at the Resection Margin Makes Lung Cancer Survivors Susceptible to SARS-CoV-2 With Unfavorable Prognosis. *Front. Oncol.* **2021**, *11*, 644575.

51. Gottschalk, G.; Knox, K.; Roy, A. ACE2: At the crossroad of COVID-19 and lung cancer. *Gene Rep.* **2021**, *23*, 101077. [CrossRef]
52. Ren, P.; Gong, C.; Ma, S. Evaluation of COVID-19 based on ACE2 expression in normal and cancer patients. *Open Med. (Wars)* **2020**, *15*, 613–622. [CrossRef]
53. Wang, H.; Yang, J. Colorectal Cancer that Highly Express Both ACE2 and TMPRSS2, Suggesting Severe Symptoms to SARS-CoV-2 Infection. *Pathol. Oncol. Res.* **2021**, *27*, 612969. [CrossRef] [PubMed]
54. Liu, C.; Wang, K.; Zhang, M.; Hu, X.; Hu, T.; Liu, Y.; Hu, Q.; Wu, S.; Yue, J. High expression of ACE2 and TMPRSS2 and clinical characteristics of COVID-19 in colorectal cancer patients. *NPJ Precis. Oncol.* **2021**, *5*, 1. [CrossRef] [PubMed]
55. Lee, S.C.; Son, K.J.; Han, C.H.; Park, S.C.; Jung, J.Y. Impact of COPD on COVID-19 prognosis: A nationwide population-based study in South Korea. *Sci. Rep.* **2021**, *11*, 3735. [CrossRef]
56. Gerayeli, F.V.; Milne, S.; Cheung, C.; Li, X.; Yang, C.W.T.; Tam, A.; Choi, L.H.; Bae, A.; Sin, D.D. COPD and the risk of poor outcomes in COVID-19: A systematic review and meta-analysis. *EClinicalMedicine* **2021**, *33*, 100789. [CrossRef]
57. Cai, G.; Bosse, Y.; Xiao, F.; Kheradmand, F.; Amos, C.I. Tobacco Smoking Increases the Lung Gene Expression of ACE2, the Receptor of SARS-CoV-2. *Am. J. Respir. Crit. Care Med.* **2020**, *201*, 1557–1559. [CrossRef] [PubMed]
58. Jacobs, M.; Van Eeckhoutte, H.P.; Wijnant, S.R.A.; Janssens, W.; Joos, G.F.; Brusselle, G.G.; Bracke, K.R. Increased expression of ACE2, the SARS-CoV-2 entry receptor, in alveolar and bronchial epithelium of smokers and COPD subjects. *Eur. Respir. J.* **2020**, *56*. [CrossRef] [PubMed]
59. Leung, J.M.; Yang, C.X.; Tam, A.; Shaipanich, T.; Hackett, T.L.; Singhera, G.K.; Dorscheid, D.R.; Sin, D.D. ACE-2 expression in the small airway epithelia of smokers and COPD patients: Implications for COVID-19. *Eur. Respir. J.* **2020**, *55*. [CrossRef]
60. Sharif-Askari, N.S.; Sharif-Askari, F.S.; Alabed, M.; Temsah, M.-H.; Al Heialy, S.; Hamid, Q.; Halwani, R. Airways Expression of SARS-CoV-2 Receptor, ACE2, and TMPRSS2 Is Lower in Children Than Adults and Increases with Smoking and COPD. *Mol. Ther. Methods Clin. Dev.* **2020**, *18*, 1–6. [CrossRef]
61. Fliesser, E.; Birnhuber, A.; Marsh, L.M.; Gschwandtner, E.; Klepetko, W.; Olschewski, H.; Kwapiszewska, G. Dysbalance of ACE2 levels—A possible cause for severe COVID-19 outcome in COPD. *J. Pathol. Clin. Res.* **2021**, *7*, 446–458. [CrossRef]
62. Council, E.-E.; Group, E.W. Chronic kidney disease is a key risk factor for severe COVID-19: A call to action by the ERA-EDTA. *Nephrol. Dial. Transplant.* **2021**, *36*, 87–94. [CrossRef]
63. Danilczyk, U.; Penninger, J.M. Angiotensin-converting enzyme II in the heart and the kidney. *Circ. Res.* **2006**, *98*, 463–471. [CrossRef] [PubMed]
64. Domenig, O.; Manzel, A.; Grobe, N.; Konigshausen, E.; Kaltenecker, C.C.; Kovarik, J.J.; Stegbauer, J.; Gurley, S.B.; van Oyen, D.; Antlanger, M.; et al. Neprilysin is a Mediator of Alternative Renin-Angiotensin-System Activation in the Murine and Human Kidney. *Sci. Rep.* **2016**, *6*, 33678. [CrossRef]
65. Kaltenecker, C.C.; Domenig, O.; Kopecky, C.; Antlanger, M.; Poglitsch, M.; Berlakovich, G.; Kain, R.; Stegbauer, J.; Rahman, M.; Hellinger, R.; et al. Critical Role of Neprilysin in Kidney Angiotensin Metabolism. *Circ. Res.* **2020**, *127*, 593–606. [CrossRef] [PubMed]
66. Maksimowski, N.; Williams, V.R.; Scholey, J.W. Kidney ACE2 expression: Implications for chronic kidney disease. *PLoS ONE* **2020**, *15*, e0241534. [CrossRef]
67. Velez, J.C.Q.; Caza, T.; Larsen, C.P. COVAN is the new HIVAN: The re-emergence of collapsing glomerulopathy with COVID-19. *Nat. Rev. Nephrol.* **2020**, *16*, 565–567. [CrossRef] [PubMed]
68. Driggin, E.; Madhavan, M.V.; Bikdeli, B.; Chuich, T.; Laracy, J.; Biondi-Zoccai, G.; Brown, T.S.; Der Nigoghossian, C.; Zidar, D.A.; Haythe, J.; et al. Cardiovascular Considerations for Patients, Health Care Workers, and Health Systems During the COVID-19 Pandemic. *J. Am. Coll. Cardiol.* **2020**, *75*, 2352–2371. [CrossRef] [PubMed]
69. Robinson, F.A.; Mihealsick, R.P.; Wagener, B.M.; Hanna, P.; Poston, M.D.; Efimov, I.R.; Shivkumar, K.; Hoover, D.B. Role of angiotensin-converting enzyme 2 and pericytes in cardiac complications of COVID-19 infection. *Am. J. Physiol. Heart Circ. Physiol.* **2020**, *319*, H1059–H1068. [CrossRef]
70. Khoury, E.E.; Knaney, Y.; Fokra, A.; Kinaneh, S.; Azzam, Z.; Heyman, S.N.; Abassi, Z. Pulmonary, cardiac and renal distribution of ACE2, furin, TMPRSS2 and ADAM17 in rats with heart failure: Potential implication for COVID-19 disease. *J. Cell. Mol. Med.* **2021**, *25*, 3840–3855. [CrossRef] [PubMed]
71. Chen, L.; Li, X.; Chen, M.; Feng, Y.; Xiong, C. The ACE2 expression in human heart indicates new potential mechanism of heart injury among patients infected with SARS-CoV-2. *Cardiovasc. Res.* **2020**, *116*, 1097–1100. [CrossRef] [PubMed]
72. Tucker, N.R.; Chaffin, M.; Bedi, K.C., Jr.; Papangeli, I.; Akkad, A.D.; Arduini, A.; Hayat, S.; Eraslan, G.; Muus, C.; Bhattacharyya, R.P.; et al. Myocyte-Specific Upregulation of ACE2 in Cardiovascular Disease: Implications for SARS-CoV-2-Mediated Myocarditis. *Circulation* **2020**, *142*, 708–710. [CrossRef]
73. Nicin, L.; Abplanalp, W.T.; Mellentin, H.; Kattih, B.; Tombor, L.; John, D.; Schmitto, J.D.; Heineke, J.; Emrich, F.; Arsalan, M.; et al. Cell type-specific expression of the putative SARS-CoV-2 receptor ACE2 in human hearts. *Eur. Heart J.* **2020**, *41*, 1804–1806. [CrossRef]
74. Popkin, B.M.; Du, S.; Green, W.D.; Beck, M.A.; Algaith, T.; Herbst, C.H.; Alsukait, R.F.; Alluhidan, M.; Alazemi, N.; Shekar, M. Individuals with obesity and COVID-19: A global perspective on the epidemiology and biological relationships. *Obes. Rev.* **2020**, *21*, e13128. [CrossRef] [PubMed]

75. Luo, H.; Wang, X.; Chen, C.; Wang, J.; Zou, X.; Li, C.; Xu, Z.; Yang, X.; Shi, W.; Zeng, C. Oxidative stress causes imbalance of renal renin angiotensin system (RAS) components and hypertension in obese Zucker rats. *J. Am. Heart. Assoc.* **2015**, *4*, e001559. [CrossRef]
76. Walls, A.C.; Park, Y.J.; Tortorici, M.A.; Wall, A.; McGuire, A.T.; Veesler, D. Structure, Function, and Antigenicity of the SARS-CoV-2 Spike Glycoprotein. *Cell* **2020**, *181*, 281–292.e6.
77. Al-Benna, S. Association of high level gene expression of ACE2 in adipose tissue with mortality of COVID-19 infection in obese patients. *Obes. Med.* **2020**, *19*, 100283. [CrossRef] [PubMed]
78. Heialy, A.S.; Hachim, M.Y.; Senok, A.; Gaudet, M.; Abou Tayoun, A.; Hamoudi, R.; Alsheikh-Ali, A.; Hamid, Q. Regulation of Angiotensin- Converting Enzyme 2 in Obesity: Implications for COVID-19. *Front. Physiol.* **2020**, *11*, 555039. [CrossRef]
79. Engeli, S.; Bohnke, J.; Gorzelniak, K.; Janke, J.; Schling, P.; Bader, M.; Luft, F.C.; Sharma, A.M. Weight loss and the renin-angiotensin-aldosterone system. *Hypertension* **2005**, *45*, 356–362. [CrossRef]
80. Rao, S.; Lau, A.; So, H.C. Exploring Diseases/Traits and Blood Proteins Causally Related to Expression of ACE2, the Putative Receptor of SARS-CoV-2: A Mendelian Randomization Analysis Highlights Tentative Relevance of Diabetes-Related Traits. *Diabetes Care* **2020**, *43*, 1416–1426. [CrossRef]
81. Batchu, S.N.; Kaur, H.; Yerra, V.G.; Advani, S.L.; Kabir, M.G.; Liu, Y.; Klein, T.; Advani, A. Lung and Kidney ACE2 and TMPRSS2 in Renin-Angiotensin System Blocker-Treated Comorbid Diabetic Mice Mimicking Host Factors That Have Been Linked to Severe COVID-19. *Diabetes* **2021**, *70*, 759–771. [CrossRef] [PubMed]
82. Wijnant, S.R.A.; Jacobs, M.; Van Eeckhoutte, H.P.; Lapauw, B.; Joos, G.F.; Bracke, K.R.; Brusselle, G.G. Expression of ACE2, the SARS-CoV-2 Receptor, in Lung Tissue of Patients With Type 2 Diabetes. *Diabetes* **2020**, *69*, 2691–2699. [CrossRef]
83. Kates, O.S.; Haydel, B.M.; Florman, S.S.; Rana, M.M.; Chaudhry, Z.S.; Ramesh, M.S.; Safa, K.; Kotton, C.N.; Blumberg, E.A.; Besharatian, B.D.; et al. COVID-19 in solid organ transplant: A multi-center cohort study. *Clin. Infect. Dis.* **2020**. Available online: https://scholarlycommons.henryford.com/infectiousdiseases_articles/126/ (accessed on 1 July 2021).
84. Heldman, M.R.; Kates, O.S. COVID-19 in Solid Organ Transplant Recipients: A Review of the Current Literature. *Curr. Treat. Options Infect. Dis.* **2021**, *13*, 67–82. [CrossRef]
85. Bottio, T.; Bagozzi, L.; Fiocco, A.; Nadali, M.; Caraffa, R.; Bifulco, O.; Ponzoni, M.; Lombardi, C.M.; Metra, M.; Russo, C.F.; et al. COVID-19 in Heart Transplant Recipients: A Multicenter Analysis of the Northern Italian Outbreak. *JACC Heart Fail.* **2021**, *9*, 52–61. [CrossRef]
86. Kovarik, J.J.; Kaltenecker, C.C.; Kopecky, C.; Domenig, O.; Antlanger, M.; Werzowa, J.; Eskandary, F.; Kain, R.; Poglitsch, M.; Schmaldienst, S.; et al. Intrarenal Renin-Angiotensin-System Dysregulation after Kidney Transplantation. *Sci. Rep.* **2019**, *9*, 9762. [CrossRef] [PubMed]
87. Soler, M.J.; Batlle, M.; Riera, M.; Campos, B.; Ortiz-Perez, J.T.; Anguiano, L.; Roca-Ho, H.; Farrero, M.; Mont, L.; Pascual, J.; et al. ACE2 and ACE in acute and chronic rejection after human heart transplantation. *Int. J. Cardiol.* **2019**, *275*, 59–64. [CrossRef] [PubMed]
88. Wysocki, J.; Lores, E.; Ye, M.; Soler, M.J.; Batlle, D. Kidney and Lung ACE2 Expression after an ACE Inhibitor or an Ang II Receptor Blocker: Implications for COVID-19. *J. Am. Soc. Nephrol.* **2020**, *31*, 1941–1943. [CrossRef]
89. Milne, S.; Yang, C.X.; Timens, W.; Bosse, Y.; Sin, D.D. SARS-CoV-2 receptor ACE2 gene expression and RAAS inhibitors. *Lancet Respir. Med.* **2020**, *8*, e50–e51. [CrossRef]
90. Jiang, X.; Eales, J.M.; Scannali, D.; Nazgiewicz, A.; Prestes, P.; Maier, M.; Denniff, M.; Xu, X.; Saluja, S.; Cano-Gamez, E.; et al. Hypertension and renin-angiotensin system blockers are not associated with expression of angiotensin-converting enzyme 2 (ACE2) in the kidney. *Eur. Heart J.* **2020**, *41*, 4580–4588. [CrossRef] [PubMed]
91. Trump, S.; Lukassen, S.; Anker, M.S.; Chua, R.L.; Liebig, J.; Thurmann, L.; Corman, V.M.; Binder, M.; Loske, J.; Klasa, C.; et al. Hypertension delays viral clearance and exacerbates airway hyperinflammation in patients with COVID-19. *Nat. Biotechnol.* **2020**. [CrossRef]
92. Lee, I.T.; Nakayama, T.; Wu, C.T.; Goltsev, Y.; Jiang, S.; Gall, P.A.; Liao, C.K.; Shih, L.C.; Schurch, C.M.; McIlwain, D.R.; et al. ACE2 localizes to the respiratory cilia and is not increased by ACE inhibitors or ARBs. *Nat. Commun.* **2020**, *11*, 5453. [CrossRef] [PubMed]
93. Patel, V.B.; Bodiga, S.; Fan, D.; Das, S.K.; Wang, Z.; Wang, W.; Basu, R.; Zhong, J.; Kassiri, Z.; Oudit, G.Y. Cardioprotective effects mediated by angiotensin II type 1 receptor blockade and enhancing angiotensin 1-7 in experimental heart failure in angiotensin-converting enzyme 2-null mice. *Hypertension* **2012**, *59*, 1195–1203. [CrossRef]
94. Wilcox, C.S.; Pitt, B. Is Spironolactone the Preferred Renin-Angiotensin-Aldosterone Inhibitor for Protection Against COVID-19? *J. Cardiovasc. Pharmacol.* **2020**, *77*, 323–331. [CrossRef]
95. Li, F.; Han, M.; Dai, P.; Xu, W.; He, J.; Tao, X.; Wu, Y.; Tong, X.; Xia, X.; Guo, W.; et al. Distinct mechanisms for TMPRSS2 expression explain organ-specific inhibition of SARS-CoV-2 infection by enzalutamide. *Nat. Commun.* **2021**, *12*, 866. [CrossRef] [PubMed]
96. Ko, C.J.; Hsu, T.W.; Wu, S.R.; Lan, S.W.; Hsiao, T.F.; Lin, H.Y.; Lin, H.H.; Tu, H.F.; Lee, C.F.; Huang, C.C.; et al. Inhibition of TMPRSS2 by HAI-2 reduces prostate cancer cell invasion and metastasis. *Oncogene* **2020**, *39*, 5950–5963. [CrossRef] [PubMed]
97. Tomita, Y.; Matsuyama, S.; Fukuhara, H.; Maenaka, K.; Kataoka, H.; Hashiguchi, T.; Takeda, M. The Physiological TMPRSS2 Inhibitor HAI-2 Alleviates SARS-CoV-2 Infection. *J. Virol.* **2021**, *95*, e00434-21. [CrossRef]

98. Chen, Y.; Lear, T.B.; Evankovich, J.W.; Larsen, M.B.; Lin, B.; Alfaras, I.; Kennerdell, J.R.; Salminen, L.; Camarco, D.P.; Lockwood, K.C. A high-throughput screen for TMPRSS2 expression identifies FDA-approved compounds that can limit SARS-CoV-2 entry. *Nat. Commun.* **2021**, *12*, 3907. [CrossRef] [PubMed]
99. Hu, X.; Shrimp, J.H.; Guo, H.; Xu, M.; Chen, C.Z.; Zhu, W.; Zakharov, A.V.; Jain, S.; Shinn, P.; Simeonov, A.; et al. Discovery of TMPRSS2 Inhibitors from Virtual Screening as a Potential Treatment of COVID-19. *ACS Pharmacol. Transl. Sci.* **2021**, *4*, 1124–1135. [CrossRef]

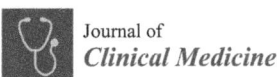

Article

Check the Need–Prevalence and Outcome after Transvenous Cardiac Implantable Electric Device Extraction without Reimplantation

Giuseppe D'Angelo [1,†], David Zweiker [1,2,3,*,†], Nicolai Fierro [1], Alessandra Marzi [1], Gabriele Paglino [1], Simone Gulletta [1], Mario Matta [4], Francesco Melillo [5], Caterina Bisceglia [1], Luca Rosario Limite [1], Manuela Cireddu [1], Pasquale Vergara [1], Francesco Bosica [1], Giulio Falasconi [1], Luigi Pannone [1], Luigia Brugliera [6], Teresa Oloriz [7], Simone Sala [1], Andrea Radinovic [1], Francesca Baratto [1], Lorenzo Malatino [8], Giovanni Peretto [1], Kenzaburo Nakajima [1], Michael D. Spartalis [1], Antonio Frontera [1], Paolo Della Bella [1] and Patrizio Mazzone [1]

1 Department of Cardiac Electrophysiology and Arrhythmology, IRCCS San Raffaele Scientific Institute, San Raffaele Hospital, Vita-Salute University, 20132 Milan, Italy; d'angelo.giuseppe@hsr.it (G.D.); fierro.nicolai@hsr.it (N.F.); marzi.alessandra@hsr.it (A.M.); paglino.gabriele@hsr.it (G.P.); gulletta.simone@hsr.it (S.G.); bisceglia.caterina@hsr.it (C.B.); lucalimite@gmail.com (L.R.L.); cireddu.manuela@hsr.it (M.C.); vergara.pasquale@hsr.it (P.V.); bosica.francesco@hsr.it (F.B.); giuliofalasconi@gmail.com (G.F.); pannone.luigi@hsr.it (L.P.); sala.simone@hsr.it (S.S.); radinovic.andrea@hsr.it (A.R.); baratto.francesca@hsr.it (F.B.); peretto.giovanni@hsr.it (G.P.); kenzabunakajima@gmail.com (K.N.); msparta@med.uoa.gr (M.D.S.); frontera.antonio@hsr.it (A.F.); dellabella.paolo@hsr.it (P.D.B.); mazzone.patrizio@hsr.it (P.M.)
2 Third Clinical Department for Cardiology and Intensive Care, Klinik Ottakring, 1160 Vienna, Austria
3 Division of Cardiology, Medical University of Graz, 8036 Graz, Austria
4 Division of Cardiology, Sant'Andrea Hospital, 13100 Vercelli, Italy; m.matta26@gmail.com
5 Department of Cardiovascular Imaging Unit, IRCCS San Raffaele Scientific Institute, San Raffaele Hospital, Vita-Salute University, 20132 Milan, Italy; francescomelillo1989@gmail.com
6 Department of Rehabilitation and Functional Recovery, IRCCS San Raffaele Scientific Institute, Vita-Salute University, 20132 Milan, Italy; brugliera.luigia@hsr.it
7 Department of Cardiology, Hospital Universitario Clínico de Zaragoza, 50009 Zaragoza, Spain; toloriz@hotmail.com
8 Department of Clinical and Experimental Medicine, University of Catania, 95131 Catania, Italy; malatino@unict.it
* Correspondence: davidzweiker@gmail.com; Tel.: +43-664-8650460
† Contributed equally.

Abstract: Background: after transvenous lead extraction (TLE) of cardiac implantable electric devices (CIEDs), some patients may not benefit from device reimplantation. This study sought to analyse predictors and long-term outcome of patients after TLE with vs. without reimplantation in a high-volume centre. Methods: all patients undergoing TLE at our centre between January 2010 and November 2015 were included into this analysis. Results: a total of 223 patients (median age 70 years, 22.0% female) were included into the study. Cardiac resynchronization therapy-defibrillator (CRT-D) was the most common device (40.4%) followed by pacemaker (PM) (31.4%), implantable cardioverter-defibrillator (ICD) (26.9%), and cardiac resynchronization therapy-PM (CRT-P) (1.4%). TLE was performed due to infection (55.6%), malfunction (35.9%), system upgrade (6.7%) or other causes (1.8%). In 14.8%, no reimplantation was performed after TLE. At a median follow-up of 41 months, no preventable arrhythmia-related events were documented in the no-reimplantation group, but 11.8% received a new CIED after 17–84 months. While there was no difference in short-term survival, five-year survival was significantly lower in the no-reimplantation group (78.3% vs. 94.7%, $p = 0.014$). Conclusions: in patients undergoing TLE, a re-evaluation of the indication for reimplantation is safe and effective. Reimplantation was not related to preventable arrhythmia events, but all-cause survival was lower.

Keywords: extraction; reimplantation; pacing; ICD; CRT

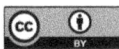

1. Introduction

Cardiovascular implantable electronic devices (CIED) are increasingly used for the treatment of brady- and tachy-arrhythmic cardiomyopathies, leading to rising numbers of patients with CIEDs [1]. However, the incidence of CIED-related complications is not negligible and in some situations transvenous lead extraction (TLE) is indicated. Infection is the most feared complication, with an incidence of 1.9 per 1000 device-years [2], being responsible for relevant morbidity and potentially life-threatening complications [2,3]. Other indications for TLE include lead failure associated with adverse arrhythmic effects, vein stenosis/occlusion, presence of recalled leads, or facilitation of MRI conditionality. Furthermore, lead extraction may be considered after shared-decision making with the patient, for example during device upgrade [2].

TLE carries a non-negligible risk of procedure-related complications, such as cardiac tamponade, tricuspid valve regurgitation, embolization, vascular complications, and death [4]. Moreover, reimplantation of CIEDs after extraction puts the patient at risk of repeat infection or complications. For this reason, current guidelines recommend patients' re-evaluation after explant, aiming to identify patients strictly requiring device reimplantation and those who can benefit from a conservative management [2,3].

The aim of this study was to identify patients without reimplantation, to assess their long-term outcome compared to remaining patients and to document the risk of further device-related complications in reimplantation patients in a high-volume tertiary centre.

2. Materials and Methods

This study is a retrospective analysis of all patients undergoing TLE at the Department of Cardiac Electrophysiology and Arrhythmology, San Raffaele Hospital, Milan, Italy, between January 2010 and November 2015. The institutional ethics committee approved the analysis.

2.1. TLE and Post-Procedural Management

The indication of TLE was set according to current guidelines [2,3] after detailed discussion with the referring physician and the patient. All TLE procedures were performed in the electrophysiology laboratory under conscious sedation or general anaesthesia using a stepwise approach as described elsewhere [4]. All lead extractions were performed with standby cardiac surgery on-site. In case of pacemaker dependency, a standard active-fixation lead was placed in the right ventricle and connected to a temporary pacemaker by the end of the procedure.

After the procedure, patients were treated in our arrhythmia unit with continuous ECG monitoring and transthoracic echocardiography was performed.

2.2. Decision to Reimplant

The decision to reimplant the CIED was based on the individual indication for new CIED implantation at time of TLE according to current international guidelines [5,6], taking into account the patient's history, clinical evaluation, frailty, Holter ECG, and echocardiogram. Second level exams, such as invasive electrophysiological study or cardiac magnetic resonance, were performed in selected patients, according to the clinical presentation. The patient's preference was especially taken into account if the indication for CIED implantation was unclear (e.g., IIb indication for implantation) or the patient strongly denied or favoured reimplantation. Pacing-dependent patients were always implanted a new CIED, but the type of device was also reassessed before reimplantation. The main indications for reimplant in pacemaker patients were intermittent or chronic high-grade AV block or symptomatic sick sinus syndrome. In patients with previous bradycardia-tachycardia syndrome, the cardiac rhythm in the year before TLE was assessed from the CIED storage and a reimplant was omitted if the patients had been in stable atrial fibrillation without episodes of bradycardia. In previous ICD patients, reimplantation was offered in patients with a history of sustained ventricular arrhythmia and a left ventricular ejection fraction below 35%. In patients with CRT, reimplant was recommended in patients with good response to CRT therapy.

The reimplantation was performed at the ipsilateral side, directly after the lead extraction, or after at least 7 days of antimicrobial therapy and negative blood cultures, for at least 72 h at the contralateral side in patients with device infection. In selected cases without the dependency of pacing, the reimplantation was performed during a second stay in hospital a few weeks after the index procedure.

2.3. Follow-Up

Following reimplantation or decision to discontinue device therapy, patients were discharged and followed thereafter in our clinic after one month and at a 6–12-month interval afterwards.

2.4. Data Collection

All patients receiving TLE at our centre were identified using the department's prospective TLE registry. Patients were excluded if the decision to reimplant was left to the referring centre and in case of in-hospital death before the decision was made. In case of multiple extractions, the first procedure was included as index procedure. Baseline, procedural and follow-up data, as well as complications, were retrieved from the hospital's information system. In case of missing follow-up, patients without reimplantation were additionally contacted via telephone.

2.5. Endpoints

Complete procedural success was defined as the removal of all targeted leads and all lead material from the vascular space without the occurrence of any permanently disabling complication or procedure-related death. Clinical success was defined as the removal of all targeted leads and lead material from the vascular space that could oppose a risk of perforation, embolic events, or perpetuation of infection, in the absence of complications. Failure of the procedure was defined as the inability to achieve either complete procedural or clinical success, or the occurrence of any permanently disabling complication, or procedure-related death. Major complications were defined as outcomes that were life-threatening, resulting in significant or permanent disability or death, or required surgical intervention. Minor complications were defined as events related to the procedure that required medical intervention or minor surgery. Device-related complication at follow-up was defined any complication that was exclusively caused by the implanted device and required invasive interventions as result; pocket changes due to battery depletion were excluded.

2.6. Statistics

Patients were stratified into two groups based on reimplantation after TLE: All patients that received reimplantation during the index stay or were scheduled a reimplantation procedure at the time of discharge were summarised into the "reimplantation" group, whereas remaining patients formed the "no reimplantation" group. Continuous variables are reported as mean (standard deviation, SD) or median (interquartile range, IQR), and categorical variables as percentage (absolute number). Continuous data were compared by student's T test or Mann-Whitney U-test as appropriate; categorical variables were compared with Fisher's test. Multivariable analysis using logistic regression analysis was performed to assess the role of predictors of the absence of need for device reimplantation. Therefore, all baseline characteristics, as shown in Table 1 with a univariable p value < 0.1, were included. A two-tailed p value < 0.05 was considered statistically significant. All analyses were performed using R 4.0.5 (The R Project, Vienna, Austria).

Table 1. Baseline characteristics of the included population.

	Total Population (n = 223)	Reimplantation (n = 190)	No Reimplantation (n = 33)	p-Value
Demographics				
Age (years)	70 (58–76)	70 (58–76)	73 (57–78)	0.703
Female gender	22.0% (n = 49)	23.2% (n = 44)	15.2% (n = 5)	0.369
Comorbidities				
Hypertension	53.4% (n = 119)	52.6% (n = 100)	57.6% (n = 19)	0.706
Diabetes mellitus	22.0% (n = 49)	20.5% (n = 39)	30.3% (n = 10)	0.254
eGFR	69.7 ± 27.7	68.7 ± 27.2	75.3 ± 30.0	0.245
eGFR < 60 mL/min	37.7% (n = 84)	38.4% (n = 73)	33.3% (n = 11)	0.698
LVEF				
35–50%	28.7% (n = 64)	29.0% (n = 55)	27.3% (n = 9)	0.043
<35%	34.5% (n = 77)	37.4% (n = 71)	18.2% (n = 6)	
Atrial fibrillation				
paroxysmal	22.9% (n = 51)	22.1% (n = 42)	27.3% (n = 9)	0.613
permanent	11.7% (n = 26)	11.1% (n = 21)	1.52% (n = 5)	
Anticoagulation	31.4% (n = 70)	32.1% (n = 61)	27.3% (n = 9)	0.686
Antiplatelets	33.2% (n = 74)	34.7% (n = 66)	24.2% (n = 8)	0.317
Device details				
Device type				
CRT-D	40.4% (n = 90)	41.6% (n = 79)	33.3% (n = 11)	0.590
PM	31.4% (n = 70)	31.6% (n = 60)	30.3% (n = 10)	
ICD	26.9% (n = 60)	25.3% (n = 48)	36.4% (n = 12)	
CRT-P	1.4% (n = 3)	1.6% (n = 3)	0% (n = 0)	
Indication for implant				
Non-ischemic CMP	38.1% (n = 85)	37.9% (n = 72)	39.4% (n = 13)	0.004
Ischemic CMP	29.6% (n = 66)	32.1% (n = 61)	15.2% (n = 5)	
AV block	12.6% (n = 28)	14.2% (n = 27)	3.0% (n = 1)	
Sick sinus syndrome	11.2% (n = 25)	8.4% (n = 16)	27.3% (n = 9)	
Inherited cardiac disease	5.4% (n = 12)	4.7% (n = 9)	9.1% (n = 3)	
other	3.1% (n = 7)	2.6% (n = 5)	6.1% (n = 2)	
Implant for secondary prevention [†]	15.5% (n= 16)	17.2% (n = 15)	6.3% (n = 1)	0.456
Indication for explant				
infection	55.6% (n = 124)	51.1% (n = 97)	81.8% (n = 27)	0.003
malfunction	35.9% (n = 80)	39.5% (n = 75)	15.2% (n = 5)	
system upgrade	6.7% (n = 15)	7.9% (n = 15)	0% (n = 0)	
other causes	1.8% (n = 4)	1.6% (n = 3)	3.0% (n = 1)	
Number of leads	2 (2–3)	2 (2–3)	2 (2–3)	0.943
Number of leads to be removed	2 (1–3)	2 (1–3)	2 (2–3)	0.033
Age of device (months)	54 (21–85)	50 (21–84)	68 (20–92)	0.633
Age of leads (months)	68 (31–100)	62 (30–99)	78 (45–104)	0.432

AV: atrioventricular; eGFR: estimated glomerular filtration rate calculated with CKD-EPI formula; LVEF: left ventricular ejection fraction; ICD: implantable cardioverter defibrillator; CMP: cardiomyopathy; CRT-D: cardiac resynchronization therapy-defibrillator; CRT-P: cardiac resynchronization therapy-pacemaker; PM: pacemaker; [†] secondary prevention as indication for primary CIED implantation in ICD and CRT-D patients (data available in 69% of cases).

3. Results

Out of 242 patients undergoing 246 TLE procedures during the observation period, 223 patients were included into the analysis. Remaining patients either died in hospital (n = 2) or the decision to reimplant was not documented or left to the referring hospital (n = 17).

3.1. Baseline Characteristics and TLE Procedure

Median age was 70 (IQR 58–76) years and 22.0% were female. Main comorbidities were reduced left ventricular ejection fraction (63.2%), arterial hypertension (53.4%), chronic kidney disease (37.7%), and atrial fibrillation (34.6%, Table 1).

Overall, 40.4% of patients had a CRT-D, 31.4% a single or dual chamber pacemaker, and 26.9% an ICD. Remaining patients had a CRT-P (1.4%).

Infection was the main reason of extraction (55.6%), which was present in the pocket in 41.3%, while systemic infection with active endocarditis was identified in 16.1%. Lead malfunction was the cause of extraction in 35.9% of patients, followed by device upgrade (6.7%) and other causes (1.8%, such as patient discomfort, Table 1). Out of 2.5 ± 0.9 present leads per patient, 2.2 ± 1.1 were planned to be explanted; an explant of the entire system was planned in 78.0%. Median lead age was 68 months with a total range of 0 to 327 months.

TLE was clinically successful in 99.6% of cases and removal was complete in 95.5%, utilizing advanced extraction tools in 35.9% of cases. Both major and minor complications occurred in 3.1% each. Further details can be found in Supplemental Table S1.

3.2. Decision Not to Reimplant

In 34 patients (14.8%), the decision not to reimplant the CIED was taken. This included 12 patients (36.4%) that previously had an ICD, 11 patients (33.3%) with CRT-D and 10 patients (30.3%) with a pacemaker. The decision was based on a negative electrophysiological study in 21.2%, restoration of LV function in 21.2%, absence of arrhythmia during continuous ECG monitoring in 18.2%, patients' preference in 12.1% and negative MRI in 6.1%. Persistent infection was another factor that played a role in the decision in 33.3% of cases. Another reason was negative electro-anatomical mapping in the presence of ARVD (n = 1, 3.0%). More details about patients that did not receive a reimplantation can be found in Supplemental Table S2.

In patients with reimplantation, a device upgrade was performed in 14.2%, while the device was downgraded in 9.0%. The reimplantation was performed mostly on the contralateral side (55.8%). In one case (0.5%), the reimplantation was performed with epicardial leads with the device in the abdomen.

3.3. Factors Favouring No Reimplantation

In patients without reimplantation, a reduced left ventricular ejection fraction was more prevalent (Table 1). Regarding the indication for CIED implantation, there were significant differences between groups, with sick sinus syndrome and inherited cardiac disease being more common in patients without reimplant. Device infection was significantly more common in this patient group (81.8% vs. 51.1%, p = 0.001), especially presence of endocarditis (33.3% vs. 13.2%, p = 0.008). In multivariable analysis, absence of ischemic cardiomyopathy (p = 0.047) and absence of AV block (p = 0.014) were significant predictors for absence of reimplantation, as well as high left-ventricular ejection fraction (p = 0.024, Table 2).

Table 2. Univariable and multivariable analysis assessing the role of clinical parameters in predicting the absence of reimplantation.

Parameter	p Value (Univariable)	OR (95% CI)	p Value (Multivariable)
Details regarding CIED indication			
Absence of ischemic CMP	0.062	3.1 (1.1–10.4)	0.047 *
Absence of AV block	0.089	14.6 (2.5–281.7)	0.014 *
Sick sinus syndrome	0.004 *	1.6 (0.5–5.2)	0.425
Clinical details			
LVEF (per 10% increase)	0.019 *	1.5 (1.1–2.3)	0.024 *
Details regarding CIED explant			
Absence of lead malfunction	0.006 *	2.2 (0.3–14.4)	0.416
Number of explanted leads, per lead	0.033 *	1.3 (0.8–2.2)	0.243
CIED infection	0.001 *	2.3 (0.4–18.5)	0.373

*: p < 0.05; CIED: cardiac implantable electric device; CMP: cardiomyopathy; AV: atrioventricular; LVEF: left ventricular ejection fraction; OR: odds ratio.

3.4. Follow-Up

Median follow-up duration was 42 months with no differences between groups (Table 3). While cumulative one-year mortality in patients with vs. without reimplantation was similar (98.0% vs. 100.0%), five-year mortality was significantly higher in patients with reimplantation (94.7% vs. 78.3%, $p = 0.014$, Figure 1). Hospitalizations for device revision (in the reimplantation group) or late reimplantation (in the no-reimplantation group) were similar (11.1% vs. 12.1%, $p = 0.771$)

Table 3. Follow-up.

	Reimplantation (n = 190)	No Reimplantation (n = 33)	p Value
Follow-up duration, months	44 (7–76)	23 (11–80)	0.883
1-year cumulative survival (NaR)	98.0% (131)	100.0% (23)	0.500
5-year cumulative survival (NaR)	94.7% (73)	78.3% (13)	0.014 *
late reimplantation or device revision	11.1% (n = 21)	12.1% (n = 4)	0.771
"Reimplantation"-specific events			
any device-related hospitalisation	11.1% (n = 21)	N/A	N/A
lead failure/dislocation	7.9% (n = 15)		
pocket revision	2.1% (n = 4)		
device recall	1.1% (n = 2)		
device infection	0.5% (n = 1)		
repeat extraction procedure	3.2% (n = 6)		
"No reimplantation"-specific events			
Reimplantation	N/A	12.1% (n = 4)	N/A

NaR: number at risk; *: $p < 0.05$.

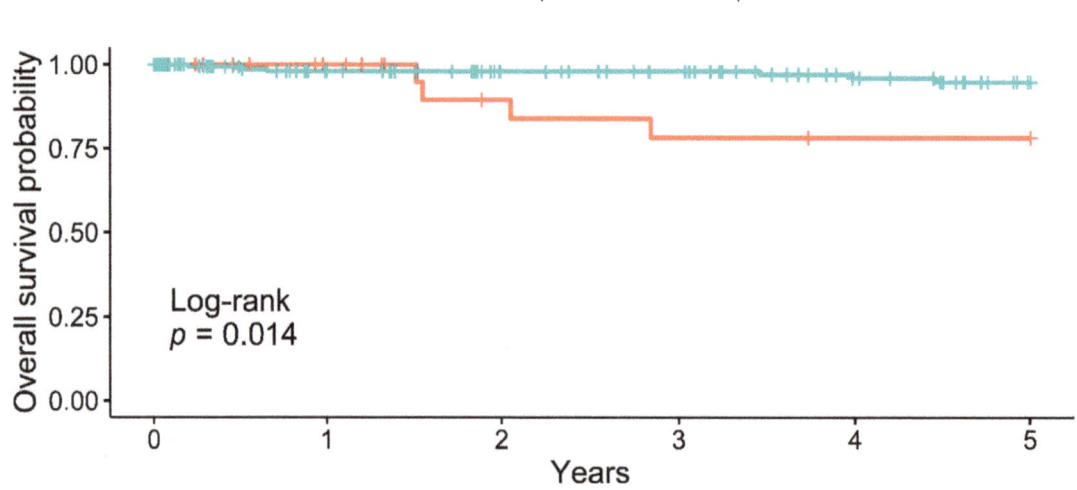

Figure 1. Cumulative survival of no-reimplantation vs. reimplantation groups.

In patients with reimplantation, device-related hospitalizations (excluding pocket changes due to battery depletion) occurred in 11.1% after an interval of 27 ± 25 months after the extraction procedure (with a range of 1 to 84 months). Reasons were lead failure necessitating repositioning (7.9%, mostly due to dislocation), pocket revision in imminent decubitus (2.1%), and generator recall (1.1%). There was one case of recurrent device infection in a female CRT-D patient that initially received extraction due of a 94-month-old fractured right ventricular lead. During follow-up after 77 months, she developed pocket dehiscence that progressed to pocket infection despite two surgical pocket revisions.

Finally, a second CIED extraction procedure was performed in six patients (3.2%) a median of 42 months after the procedure.

In patients without reimplantation, 15.2% received an implantable loop recorder for detection of pauses in two patients (6.1%) with previous PM and for detection of ventricular arrhythmias in three patients (9.1%) with previous ICD. In total, four patients (12.1%) had a late reimplantation of their device; two patients received an ICD for ventricular arrhythmias and two patients received a CRT-D reimplantation for progressing heart failure. No repeat hospitalizations for invasive treatment of recurrent infection were documented (Supplemental Table S2).

4. Discussion

This analysis of consecutive patients undergoing TLE at our centre reveals that (1) prevention of reimplantation was possible in a significant proportion of patients undergoing TLE with a low risk of arrhythmia-related events; (2) baseline comorbidities and the primary indication for CIED implantation are the main predictors for device reimplantation; and (3) long-term mortality was higher in patients without reimplantation, but mostly due to non-cardiac causes.

This study shows that following a rigorous work-up, patients that do not profit from a CIED reimplantation can be identified with a low risk of complications due to undertreatment. In this analysis, in 15.2% of cases an immediate reimplantation was prevented. Due to the heterogeneity of clinical characteristics of patients undergoing TLE, we did not identify a "one size fits all" regimen to evaluate the need for reimplantation; instead, a patient-tailored approach was necessary, including the patient's clinical status and will, cardiac magnetic resonance imaging, electrophysiologic study, and loop recorder implantation. As a CIED implantation may has a significant impact on the patient's daily life [7], the patient's opinion has to be incorporated in the final decision; it played a major role in 14.8% of cases without reimplantation in this analysis. In multiple regression analysis, we identified the CIED indication and the current left-ventricular ejection fraction to be significantly correlated with the decision to reimplantation. Patients without high degree atrioventricular block were more likely to be discharged without a CIED, probably because other indications for PM implantation have a higher potential to resolve (e.g., permanent AF in patients with previous symptomatic brady-tachy-syndrome). Patients without reimplantation were less likely to suffer from ischemic cardiomyopathy and reduced left-ventricular ejection fraction, as these conditions represent a class I indication for ICD implantation according to current guidelines [5]. In the current literature, similar (14.3%) [8] or even higher rates (40.7%) [9] of patients without reimplantation after TLE can be found. Differences in reimplantation may be explained by the incorporation of patients receiving TLE for indications other than CIED infection in this analysis. Interestingly, we did not find patients that had no indication for CIED therapy at time of implantation in contrast to Döring et al., who reported a proportion of 27% in patients without reimplantation [9].

During follow-up, we fortunately did not document a signal towards events caused by missing reimplantation in the no-reimplant group and for 17 months, no reimplantation occurred. Furthermore, we did not document ongoing device complications leading to repeat interventions in this group. Considering long-term outcome, it is apparent that more than one in ten patients out of this group may still need a reimplantation, but many years after initial TLE. Therefore, medical checks at regular intervals may be good for these patients, which is indeed more difficult considering that they do not have a CIED anymore. Interestingly, hospitalizations for CIED revision in the reimplantation group and late CIED reimplantation in the no-reimplantation group were similar.

In the whole population, there was no reintervention due to recurrent CIED infection necessary; only one patient with previous lead failure developed device infection at follow-up. The low rate of CIED reinfection is consistent with previous literature [10]. However, a significant proportion of patients with device-reimplantation (7.9%) had to be hospitalised for CIED revision, mostly due to lead dislocation. Therefore, a close follow-up may be beneficial in these patients.

While long-term survival was significantly lower in the no-reimplantation group, we did not identify deaths that may have been prevented by CIEDs. The reduced mortality in the no-reimplantation group was also seen in other studies dealing with reimplantation after TLE [8,9], but this effect is explained to be caused by older age and a high rate of non-cardiac deaths in the no-reimplantation group [9].

Limitations

While this study adds valuable evidence on the long-term outcome of patients undergoing TLE at a high-volume centre with vs. without reimplantation, it is subject to a few limitations: first, it is subject to bias (such as information bias) due to its retrospective nature. Despite rigorous investigation and telephonic contact of patients, some patients were lost to follow-up. Second, the low rate of patients may have led to underpowering of factors that explain no-reimplantation. Third, this analysis may not be extrapolated to other centres with a different volume and different TLE indications as well as procedures. Furthermore, no data about dependency on temporary pacing after TLE was available, as well as details of the primary CIED implantation (e.g., LVEF in CRT patients). Lastly, with the evolution of leadless pacing in the last years new concepts may allow the reimplantation of devices that previously was deemed too risky [11,12].

5. Conclusions

The prevention of reimplantation after TLE, after careful evaluation, is safe and does not lead to an increased rate of preventable arrhythmia-related events. The primary indication and current left-ventricular ejection fraction represent independent predictors for reimplantation. Patients without reimplantation experience reduced long-term survival compared to remaining patients at follow-up.

Supplementary Materials: The following are available online at https://www.mdpi.com/article/10.3390/jcm10184043/s1, Table S1: Procedural outcome, Table S2: Individual patient characteristics of patients without reimplantation.

Author Contributions: Conceptualization, G.D.; methodology, G.D., D.Z., P.M.; validation, G.D., D.Z., N.F., A.M., G.P. (Gabriele Paglino), S.G., M.M., F.M., L.R.L., C.B., M.C., P.V., F.B. (Francesco Bosica), G.F., L.P., L.B., T.O., S.S., A.R., F.B. (Francesca Baratto), L.M., G.P. (Giovanni Peretto), K.N., M.D.S., A.F., P.D.B., P.M.; formal analysis, G.D., D.Z.; investigation, G.D., D.Z.; resources, G.D., P.D.B., P.M.; data curation, G.D., P.M., D.Z.; writing—original draft preparation, G.D., D.Z., A.F., P.D.B., P.M.; writing—review and editing, G.D., D.Z., N.F., A.M., G.P. (Gabriele Paglino), S.G., M.M., F.M., L.R.L., C.B., M.C., P.V., F.B. (Francesco Bosica), G.F., L.P., L.B., T.O., S.S., A.R., F.B. (Francesca Baratto), L.M., G.P. (Giovanni Peretto), K.N., M.D.S., A.F., P.D.B., P.M.; visualization, D.Z.; supervision, G.D., P.M.; project administration, G.D., P.M.; funding acquisition, P.M. All authors have read and agreed to the published version of the manuscript.

Funding: This research received no external funding.

Institutional Review Board Statement: According to the institution's ethical review board, no formal ethical review was necessary for the study due to its retrospective nature.

Informed Consent Statement: Patient consent was waived due to the study's retrospective nature.

Data Availability Statement: The data presented in this study are available on request from the corresponding author.

Conflicts of Interest: D.Z. received speaker honoraria and travel grants from Daiichi Sankyo and research grants from Boston Scientific. P.M. is a proctor for Cook Medical. All other authors report no conflict of interest whatsoever.

References

1. Greenspon, A.J.; Patel, J.D.; Lau, E.; Ochoa, J.A.; Frisch, D.R.; Ho, R.T.; Pavri, B.B.; Kurtz, S.M. 16-year trends in the infection burden for pacemakers and implantable cardioverter-defibrillators in the United States 1993 to 2008. *J. Am. Coll. Cardiol.* **2011**, *58*, 1001–1006. [CrossRef] [PubMed]
2. Kusumoto, F.M.; Schoenfeld, M.H.; Wilkoff, B.L.; Berul, C.I.; Birgersdotter-Green, U.M.; Carrillo, R.; Cha, Y.M.; Clancy, J.; Deharo, J.C.; Ellenbogen, K.A.; et al. 2017 HRS expert consensus statement on cardiovascular implantable electronic device lead management and extraction. *Heart Rhythm* **2017**, *14*, e503–e551. [CrossRef] [PubMed]
3. Habib, G.; Lancellotti, P.; Antunes, M.J.; Bongiorni, M.G.; Casalta, J.P.; Del Zotti, F.; Dulgheru, R.; El Khoury, G.; Erba, P.A.; Iung, B.; et al. 2015 ESC Guidelines for the management of infective endocarditis: The Task Force for the management of infective endocarditis of the European Society of Cardiology (ESC). Endorsed by: European Association for Cardio-Thoracic Surgery (EACTS), the European Association of Nuclear Medicine (EANM). *Eur. Heart J.* **2015**, *36*, 3075–3128. [CrossRef] [PubMed]
4. Bontempi, L.; Curnis, A.; Della Bella, P.; Cerini, M.; Radinovic, A.; Inama, L.; Melillo, F.; Salghetti, F.; Marzi, A.; Gargaro, A.; et al. The MB score: A new risk stratification index to predict the need for advanced tools in lead extraction procedures. *EP Eur.* **2020**, *22*, 613–621. [CrossRef] [PubMed]
5. Ponikowski, P.; Voors, A.A.; Anker, S.D.; Bueno, H.; Cleland, J.G.; Coats, A.J.; Falk, V.; Gonzalez-Juanatey, J.R.; Harjola, V.P.; Jankowska, E.A.; et al. 2016 ESC Guidelines for the diagnosis and treatment of acute and chronic heart failure: The Task Force for the diagnosis and treatment of acute and chronic heart failure of the European Society of Cardiology (ESC)Developed with the special contribution of the Heart Failure Association (HFA) of the ESC. *Eur. Heart J.* **2016**, *37*, 2129–2200. [CrossRef] [PubMed]
6. Brignole, M.; Auricchio, A.; Baron-Esquivias, G.; Bordachar, P.; Boriani, G.; Breithardt, O.A.; Cleland, J.; Deharo, J.C.; Delgado, V.; Elliott, P.M.; et al. 2013 ESC Guidelines on cardiac pacing and cardiac resynchronization therapy: The Task Force on cardiac pacing and resynchronization therapy of the European Society of Cardiology (ESC). Developed in collaboration with the European Heart Rhythm Association (EHRA). *Eur. Heart J.* **2013**, *34*, 2281–2329. [CrossRef] [PubMed]
7. Eckert, M.; Jones, T. How does an implantable cardioverter defibrillator (ICD) affect the lives of patients and their families? *Int. J. Nurs. Pract.* **2002**, *8*, 152–157. [CrossRef] [PubMed]
8. Al-Hijji, M.A.; Killu, A.M.; Yousefian, O.; Hodge, D.O.; Park, J.Y.; Hebsur, S.; El Sabbagh, A.; Pretorius, V.G.; Ackerman, M.J.; Friedman, P.A.; et al. Outcomes of lead extraction without subsequent device reimplantation. *EP Eur.* **2017**, *19*, 1527–1534. [CrossRef] [PubMed]
9. Doring, M.; Hienzsch, L.; Ebert, M.; Lucas, J.; Dagres, N.; Kuhl, M.; Hindricks, G.; Knopp, H.; Richter, S. Extraction of infected cardiac implantable electronic devices and the need for subsequent re-implantation. *Int. J. Cardiol.* **2020**, *309*, 84–91. [CrossRef] [PubMed]
10. Boyle, T.A.; Uslan, D.Z.; Prutkin, J.M.; Greenspon, A.J.; Baddour, L.M.; Danik, S.B.; Tolosana, J.M.; Le, K.; Miro, J.M.; Peacock, J.; et al. Reimplantation and repeat infection after cardiac-implantable electronic device infections: Experience from the MEDIC (multicenter electrophysiologic device infection cohort) database. *Circ. Arrhythm. Electrophysiol.* **2017**, *10*, e004822. [CrossRef] [PubMed]
11. Kypta, A.; Blessberger, H.; Kammler, J.; Lambert, T.; Lichtenauer, M.; Brandstaetter, W.; Gabriel, M.; Steinwender, C. Leadless cardiac pacemaker implantation after lead extraction in patients with severe device infection. *J. Cardiovasc. Electrophysiol.* **2016**, *27*, 1067–1071. [CrossRef] [PubMed]
12. Gonzales, H.; Richardson, T.D.; Montgomery, J.A.; Crossley, G.H.; Ellis, C.R. Comparison of leadless pacing and temporary externalized pacing following cardiac implanted device extraction. *J. Innov. Card. Rhythm. Manag.* **2019**, *10*, 3930–3936. [CrossRef] [PubMed]

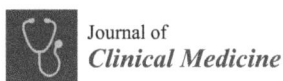

Article

Clinical Features of LMNA-Related Cardiomyopathy in 18 Patients and Characterization of Two Novel Variants

Valentina Ferradini [1], Joseph Cosma [2], Fabiana Romeo [2], Claudia De Masi [1], Michela Murdocca [1], Paola Spitalieri [1], Sara Mannucci [1], Giovanni Parlapiano [1], Francesca Di Lorenzo [1], Annamaria Martino [3], Francesco Fedele [4], Leonardo Calò [3], Giuseppe Novelli [1,5,6], Federica Sangiuolo [1,*] and Ruggiero Mango [2]

1. Department of Biomedicine and Prevention, University of Rome "Tor Vergata", 00133 Rome, Italy; ferradini@med.uniroma2.it (V.F.); claudia.dem7@gmail.com (C.D.M.); miky.murdi@hotmail.it (M.M.); paola.spitalieri@uniroma2.it (P.S.); sara.mannucci@yahoo.it (S.M.); parlapiano.giovanni@gmail.com (G.P.); francescadl1992@gmail.com (F.D.L.); novelli@med.uniroma2.it (G.N.)
2. Cardiology Unit, Department of Emergency and Critical Care, Tor Vergata Hospital, 00133 Rome, Italy; josephcosma1990@gmail.com (J.C.); fabiana.romeo87@gmail.com (F.R.); ruggiero.mango@gmail.com (R.M.)
3. Division of Cardiology, Policlinico Casilino, 00118 Rome, Italy; martinoannamaria@yahoo.it (A.M.); leonardocalo.doc@gmail.com (L.C.)
4. Department of Cardiovascular, Respiratory, Nephrology, Anesthesiology and Geriatric Sciences, Sapienza University of Rome, 00185 Rome, Italy; francesco.fedele@uniroma1.it
5. Istituto di Ricovero e Cura a Carattere Scientifico IRCCS Neuromed, Pozzilli, 86077 Isernia, Italy
6. Department of Pharmacology, School of Medicine, University of Nevada, Reno, NV 89557, USA
* Correspondence: sangiuolo@med.uniroma2.it

Abstract: Dilated cardiomyopathy (DCM) refers to a spectrum of heterogeneous myocardial disorders characterized by ventricular dilation and depressed myocardial performance in the absence of hypertension, valvular, congenital, or ischemic heart disease. Mutations in LMNA gene, encoding for lamin A/C, account for 10% of familial DCM. LMNA-related cardiomyopathies are characterized by heterogeneous clinical manifestations that vary from a predominantly structural heart disease, mainly mild-to-moderate left ventricular (LV) dilatation associated or not with conduction system abnormalities, to highly pro-arrhythmic profiles where sudden cardiac death (SCD) occurs as the first manifestation of disease in an apparently normal heart. In the present study, we select, among 77 DCM families referred to our center for genetic counselling and molecular screening, 15 patient heterozygotes for LMNA variants. Segregation analysis in the relatives evidences other eight heterozygous patients. A genotype–phenotype correlation has been performed for symptomatic subjects. Lastly, we perform in vitro functional characterization of two novel LMNA variants using dermal fibroblasts obtained from three heterozygous patients, evidencing significant differences in terms of lamin expression and nuclear morphology. Due to the high risk of SCD that characterizes patients with lamin A/C cardiomyopathy, genetic testing for LMNA gene variants is highly recommended when there is suspicion of laminopathy.

Keywords: dilated cardiomyopathy (DCM); LMNA; lamin A; lamin C; next generation sequencing (NGS)

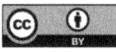

1. Introduction

Dilated cardiomyopathy (DCM) refers to a spectrum of heterogeneous myocardial disorders characterized by ventricular dilation and depressed myocardial performance in the absence of hypertension, valvular, congenital, or ischemic heart disease. Diverse aetiologies for DCM have been revealed, including genetic mutations, infections, inflammation, autoimmune diseases, exposure to toxins, and endocrine or neuromuscular causes [1]. As regards to genetic forms of DCM, more than 40 genes have been identified, causing defects in various cellular compartments and pathways such as the nuclear envelope, the contractile apparatus, the Z-disk, and calcium handling [2].

Mutations in LMNA (MIM 150330) gene, encoding for lamin A/C, account for 0.5–5% of DCM; however, its prevalence increases up to 10% in familial DCM and up to 33% in DCM associated to atrioventricular conduction disorders [3,4]. Lamin proteins form the nuclear lamina, a protein meshwork laying the inner surface of the nuclear envelope [5]. Lamin A and lamin C represents two isoforms encoded by a single gene (LMNA), located on chromosome 1q21.2-q21.3 [6]. Lamins, in addition to conferring cellular and nuclear integrity [7], are implicated in a plethora of crucial cellular functions, such as mechano-transduction, chromatin protection/organization, regulation of signaling, and gene expression [8,9]. To date, more than 500 LMNA variants have been reported [10] causing a wide variety of diseases and ranging from premature ageing to metabolic and skeletal muscle disorders [11,12].

LMNA-related cardiomyopathies are characterized by heterogeneous clinical manifestations that vary from a predominant structural heart disease, mainly mild-to-moderate left ventricular (LV) dilatation associated or not with conduction system abnormalities, to high pro-arrhythmic profile, where sudden cardiac death (SCD) occurs as first manifestation in an apparently normal heart [3]. Brady- and tachy-arrhythmias are a very common finding in lamin cardiomyopathies with conduction system disease commonly preceding the development of DCM by few years to a decade or more [13]. Moreover, supraventricular tachyarrhythmias (SVT) are generally more common than malignant ventricular arrhythmias (VA) at first clinical contact [14]. The mode of inheritance of cardiac laminopathies is autosomal dominant with an almost complete penetrance by the seventh decade [15–17]. Lamin cardiomyopathies are characterized by a poor prognosis and a high rate of major cardiac events, with the most aggressive clinical course [18].

In the present study, we report the genotype–phenotype correlation of 18 DCM patients evidenced heterozygotes for LMNA variants out of 77 referred to our Medical Genetics Unit. In three of them, functional analyses have been performed in order to validate the pathogenicity of two novel lamin variants detected during this work.

2. Materials and Methods

2.1. Study Population

Seventy-seven DCM patients and their relatives followed up at the Cardiology Unit of Policlinico Casilino (Rome, Italy) were genotyped at the Medical Genetics Unit of Tor Vergata Hospital; after genetic counselling and informed consent was signed, 15 probands evidenced heterozygotes for LMNA variants.

2.2. Clinical and Instrumental Characterization

Probands were defined as the first patients in a family referred for genetic testing due to a diagnosis of phenotypic DCM based on the Mestroni criteria for familial DCM [19]. The age of onset of symptoms or documented first traits of the disease was recorded. Family members who underwent genetic testing as part of family screening and had no reported cardiac symptoms at the time of the genetic testing were defined as genotype-positive phenotype-negative family members. Atrioventricular block by PR interval was assessed from a resting 12-lead electrocardiography (ECG). Arrhythmias (atrial and ventricular) were collected from a resting 12-lead ECG, exercise ECG, Holter monitoring and pacemaker, or implantable cardioverter defibrillator (ICD) monitoring. Ventricular arrhythmias were classified as non-sustained ventricular tachycardia (VT), defined as ≥ 3 consecutive ventricular beats with a rate ≥ 120/min lasting <30 s, or sustained VA, defined as VT with a rate ≥ 120/min lasting >30 s, ventricular fibrillation (VF), appropriate antitachycardia pacing (ATP) therapy, appropriate defibrillator shock therapy, and aborted cardiac arrest. Implantable cardioverter defibrillator and cardiac resynchronization therapy (CRT) interrogations were retrospectively reviewed and eventual therapies (ATP or defibrillator shock) recorded. Two-dimensional echocardiography was performed at the subject's first visit using the Vivid 7 or Vivid E9 system (GE Healthcare, Horten, Norway) and analyzed using commercially available software (EchoPACVR, GE). LV ejection fraction (EF) and

LV volumes were calculated from apical views using Simpson's biplane method. Left ventricular diameters were obtained from the parasternal long-axis view. When possible, patients underwent CMR at baseline by using a 1.5-T scanner (Philips Intera CV; Philips Healthcare, Best, The Netherlands) and a phased array cardiac receiver coil, according to standard acquisition protocols set by the Society for Cardiovascular Magnetic Resonance [20]. Electrocardiogram-gated, breath-hold steady-state free precession cine images were acquired in both the long- and the short-axis planes from the LV apex to the LV base. Images were subsequently analyzed offline by using a commercially available software (View Forum software, Version 5.1, Philips Healthcare, Best, The Netherlands). LV and RV end-diastolic diameters and volumes as well as end-systolic diameters and volumes, stroke volumes, EF, and left atrium area were calculated, in accordance with the Society of Cardiac Magnetic Resonance criteria [21], by using the Extended MR WorkSpace 2.6.3.4, 2012 Philips Medical System work-station. LV dilatation was diagnosed in the presence of indexed end-diastolic volumes >81 mL/m^2 for men and >76 mL/m^2 for women, respectively [22].

2.3. Genetic Analysis

Genomic DNA was extracted from peripheral blood using EZ1 AdvancedXL (Qiagen), according to the manufacturer's instructions. After Qubit 2.0 quantification, NGS was performed (Ion Torrent S5 and Ion Chef System) using a Custom Panel for SCD (Supplementary Table S1), designed by Ion Ampliseq Designer (Thermo Fisher Scientific, Waltham, MA, USA). Results were analyzed with Ion Reporter and Integrated Genome Viewer (IGV). The interpretation of genetic variants was conducted by Human Gene Mutation Database (HGMD), VarSome, ClinVar, Exac, and GnomAD. Moreover, DANN and Genomic Evolutionary Rate Profiling (GERP) were used. Sanger sequencing was used to confirm genetic variants and segregation analysis.

2.4. Fibroblasts Derivation from Skin Biopsy

Primary skin fibroblasts were obtained by a skin punch biopsy from two healthy donors (WT) and three DCM patients, after written consent. Tissues were treated as already described [23], and after 15 days, primary culture of the derived human dermal fibroblasts (HDFs) was expanded and analyzed.

2.5. Immunofluorescence

HDFs were incubated with primary antibodies anti-Lamin A/C (N-18, sc-6215, Santa Cruz Biotechnology) and anti-prelamin A (C-20, sc-6214, Santa Cruz Biotechnology), as described [23]. Nuclei were counterstained with HOECHST (33342, Thermo Fisher Scientific, Waltham, MA, USA). Images have been acquired by fluorescence microscope (Zeiss Axioplan).

2.6. Detection of Nuclear Abnormalities

For every patient's fibroblast culture, at least 3 × 100 cells in different areas of the sample were evaluated using a Zeiss Axiplan fluorescence microscope, equipped with a 100× oil objective (Plan Apo, NA1.32). Different aspects of nuclear morphology were assessed: nuclear blebs (herniations), extensive lobulations, or donut-like invaginations of the nucleus; also, Lamin staining abnormalities were scored, including extranuclear staining and the presence of so-called honeycombs. Morphometric analysis of nuclei of HDFs WT and DCM has been performed on images from Zeiss Axiplan fluorescence microscope (Hoechst-stained nuclei), using the ImageJ processing software (http://rsbweb.nih.gov/ij/ (accessed on 20 May 2020)), by analyzing at least 10 field/sample or a minimum of 300 cells/sample. The following parameters have been analyzed by tracing nuclei and obtaining, from the ImageJ software, the following parameters: (i) nucleus area, (ii) nucleus circularity (with a value of 1.0 indicating a perfect circle), (iii) nucleus elongation (aspect ratio: the major axis over the minor axis of the fit ellipse), and (iv) nucleus roundness (the inverse of aspect ratio). The analyses have been performed on images from three different experiments, and results have been reported as mean values ± SD (fold DM vs. WT). Statistical analyses have been assessed by using the Student's two-tailed t-test (* $p < 0.05$ as statistically significant).

2.7. Gene Expression Analysis

After TRIzol extraction (Invitrogen; Life Technologies Corporation, Carlsbad, CA, USA), total RNAs of patients and controls HDFs were DNase I (RNase-free)-treated (Ambion; Life Technologies Corporation), reverse transcribed using the High-Capacity cDNA Archive kit (Life Technologies Corporation) and used in real-time reverse transcription (RT)–polymerase chain reaction (PCR). mRNAs levels were measured by SYBR Green chemistry (Life Technologies Corporation) using the following primers: Lamin A: forward 5′-ACTGGGGAAGAAGTGGCCAT-3′; Lamin A: reverse 5′-GCTGCAGTGGGAGCCGT-3′; Lamin C: forward 5′-AACTCCACTGGGGAAGAAG-3′; Lamin C: reverse 5′-CATCTCCAT CCTCATGGTC-3′; GAPDH: forward 5′-TTGCCCTCAACGACCACTTTG-3′; GAPDH: reverse 5′-CACCCTGTTGCTGTAGCCAAATTC-3′. GAPDH was used as reference gene. WT value corresponds to the mean value of two wild type samples.

2.8. Western Blot Assay

Proteins were extracted from patients and controls fibroblasts by RIPA Lysis buffer and Western blot analysis performed with primary antibody for Lamin A/C (N-18, sc-6215, Santa Cruz Biotechnology), followed by Mouse anti-Goat IgG (PIERCE Biotechnology). The signals were scanned and quantified on the ImageQuant LAS 4000 system, after normalizing with f β-actin. WT value corresponds to the mean value of two wild type samples.

3. Results

3.1. Lamin A/C Variants and Cardiac Phenotype among DCM Patients

Among 77 DCM families, 11 different LMNA variants were found in 15 subjects (19.5%) and confirmed by Sanger sequencing. The segregation analysis in nineteen relatives evidenced eight heterozygotes for a total of 23 (Table 1). The remaining 62 patients evidenced heterozygotes for variants in *TTN*, *DSP*, *MYBPC3*, *MYH7*, and *SCN5A* genes.

Table 1. LMNA gene variants identified in this study.

LMNA Variant (NM_170707)	Exon	Domain	dbSNP	# Proband	# Related Individuals Carrying the Variant
E161K	2	Coil 1B	rs28933093	1 (M)	-
R189W	3	Coil 1B	rs267607626	1 (M)	-
R189Q	3	Coil 1B	rs766856162	1 (M)	1 (F)
T224I	4	Linker 2	-	1 (M)	-
R225X	4	Linker 2	rs60682848	1 (F)	-
R216H	4	Linker 2	rs757041809;/	1 (F)	-
R331L	6	Coil 2			
E317K	6	Coil 2	rs56816490	6 (5M + 1F)	5 (3M + 2F)
G382=	6	Coil 2	rs57508089	1 (M)	1 (M)
c.1381-5G > A	Intron 7		rs730880133	1 (M)	-
W467X	8	Tail	-	1 (M)	1 (M)

stands for the number of analyzed proband for each variant on LMNA gene.

Variant classification has been made applying the ACMG/AMP guidelines [24] (Table 2). Among 23 heterozygous patients, 18 (15 males and 3 females) (Table 3) referred symptoms and/or signs of DCM, while 5 subjects were asymptomatic with apparently no signs of the disease, most likely due to their young age (from 11 to 27 years old).

Table 2. Classification of LMNA variants identified.

LMNA Variant (NM_170707)	ClinVar	ACMG Classification	DANNScore	GERP	GnomAd (Allele Frequency)
E161K	Pathogenic	Likely pathogenic	0.9992	5.59	/
R189W	Uncertain significance	Likely pathogenic	0.9956	5.44	0.0000159
R189Q	Uncertain significance	Likely pathogenic	0.998	5.44	0.0000318
R216H	Uncertain significance	Likely pathogenic	0.9995	5.2699	0.0000239
T224I	/	Likely pathogenic	0.9978	5.2699	/
R225X	Pathogenic	Pathogenic	0.9974	5.2699	/
E317K	Likely pathogenic	Pathogenic	0.9992	5.67	0.0000319
R331L	/	Likely pathogenic	09987	5.67	/
G382=	Likely pathogenic/Pathogenic	Likely Pathogenic	0.7586	5.3	/
c.1381-5G > A	Uncertain significance	Uncertain significance	0.7824	5.21	0.0000482
W467X	Pathogenic	Pathogenic	0.9935	5.13	/

All variants were located within the coil domain (Figure 1), except for W467X, a non-sense variant within the tail domain. Its clinical features are very aggressive: early onset (3rd decade), LV dilation, severe reduced systolic function, large scar in the IVS and inferior wall, and complex ventricular arrhythmias. We also characterized a proband compound heterozygous (R216H/R331L) presenting worse clinical and instrumental findings. The patient (female) with onset of symptoms in the 6th decade, and severe LV systolic dysfunction (LVEF 30%), experienced supraventricular and ventricular arrhythmias, with multiple appropriate ICD shocks.

The mean age of signs/symptoms onset in 18 symptomatic patients was 51.3 ± 12.9 years. At echocardiographic examination, mean LVEDDi was 29.2 ± 4.3 mm/m2 with LVEF $42.6 \pm 10.2\%$, LA dilation was present in 15 of them (83.3%). Three patients (16.6%) had right heart involvement with RV dilation and dysfunction (CG11, CG12, and CG14). Cardiac MR performed in 15 phenotype-positive patients showed a LVEF of $46 \pm 12\%$ and generally a mild-to-moderate LV enlargement with mean LVEDVi 86 ± 32.8 mL/m2. A late gadolinium enhancement (LGE) as a sign of fibrosis was present in 13 of 15 affected subjects that underwent cardiac MR (86.6%), with interventricular septum (IVS) involvement in nine of them (69.2%). Analysis of basal ECG showed AV delay in 10 of 17 patients in sinus rhythm (58.8%) and IV delay in 9 of 18 patients (50%) (LBBB in 66.6%), a mean cQT of 420 ± 28 ms. The first clinical manifestation was ventricular arrhythmias (VA) in eight (44.5%) patients, advanced atrioventricular block in four (22.2%), and left ventricular dysfunction in six (33.3%). Twelve (66.6%) patients underwent ICD implantation: nine patients received ICD implantation before diagnosis of lamin cardiomyopathy was made because of the occurrence of ventricular arrhythmias in eight (CG02, CG03, CG05, CG06, CG07, CG09, CG10, and CG11) as secondary prevention and because of severe LV dysfunction in one (CG12) as primary prevention; two patients (CG8A and CG14A) whose onset was characterized by moderate LVEF dysfunction underwent ICD implantation once LMNA mutation was diagnosed, while in one patient (CG13), first clinical presentation was an AVB, and so a PMK was implanted, and, only after diagnosis of LMNA, an upgrade to ICD was performed. As regards patients CG8A, CG14A, and CG13, they received ICD implantation after genetic diagnosis of a LMNA variant according to the European Guidelines that suggest ICD implantation in lamin DCM if two of the following conditions are met: male sex, non-sustained VT, non-missense LMNA variant, and LVEF < 45% (patient CG8A: male sex, non-missense variant, LVEF 44%; patient CG14A: male sex, LVEF 45%; patient CG13: male sex, evidence of VA at PMK interrogation).

Table 3. DCM clinical phenotypes.

	CG01	CG02	CG03	CG04	CG05	CG06	CG07	CG08	CG08_A	CG09	CG10	CG10_A	CG11	CG12	CG13	CG14	CG14_A	CG15	Mean Value (n = 18)
LMNA variant	E317K	E317K	R189W	E317K	c.1381+5G > A	R189Q	E317K	G382=	G382=	R225X	W467X	W467X	R216H/R331L	T224I	E161K	E317K	E317K	E317K	
Biological Sex (M = 1, F = 0)	1	1	1	1	1	1	0	1	1	0	1	1	0	1	1	1	1	1	15/18 M (83.3%)
Age at Onset (years)	48	59	64	69	56	44	57	40	66	59	32	19	56	38	64	53	50	50	51.3 ± 12.9
LVEDD (mm)	65	53	52	60	64	54	50	67	57	55	57	44	54	65	51	65	51	52	56.4 ± 6.5
LVEDDi (mm/m²)	29.8	24.3	26.3	31.6	38.3	24.4	24.6	31.6	31.7	32.3	33.1	27	36.5	24.5	28.3	29.9	23.8	28.8	29.2 ± 4.3
EF echo (%)	40	55	50	37	25	51	50	35	44	53	35	50	30	20	50	45	45	51	42.6 ± 10.2
EF CMR (%)	31	69	60	46	20	55	55	37	/	50	40	51	39	/	/	42	45	50	46 ± 12
LVEDV CMR (ml)	88	99	112	247	273	151	128	243	/	158	184	138	131	/	/	172	157	150	162.1 ± 54.5
LVEDVi CMR (mL/m²)	40	45	57	130	163	68	56	115	/	87	106	85	88.5	/	/	88	79	83	86 ± 32.8
AV delay (0 = no, 1 = yes)	0	1	0	1	0	0	1	0	1	/	0	0	0	1	0	1	1	1	10/17 (58.8%)
IV delay (0 = no, 1 = yes)	1	0	/	1	0	0	0	0	1	1	0	0	1	1	1	0	1	1	9 (50%)
LBBB (0 = no, 1 = yes)	0	/	/	/	/	/	/	/	1	0	/	/	1	/	/	/	1	0	6/9 (66.6%)
AVB (0 = no, 1 = yes)	0	1	0	1	0	0	0	0	0	1	/	0	0	0	1	0	0	1	6 (33.3%)
cQT (msec)	430	395	408	430	428	386	400	420	425	490	400	392	470	440	390	421	438	400	420 ± 28
LA dilatation (0 = no, 1 = yes)	1	1	1	1	1	1	1	1	0	1	1	0	1	1	1	1	1	1	15 (83.3%)
RV involvement (0 = no, 1 = yes)	0	0	0	0	1	0	0	0	0	0	0	0	1	1	0	0	0	0	3 (16.6%)
CMR scar (0 = no, 1 = yes)	1	1	1	0	1	1	0	1	/	1	1	1	1	/	/	1	1	1	13/15 (86.6%)
Scar IVS involvement (0 = no, 1 = yes)	0	1	1	/	1	0	/	1	/	1	1	0	1	/	/	0	1	1	9/13 (69.2)
First clinical manifestation (VA = 1, AVB = 2, LV dysfunction = 3)	3	1	1	2	1	1	1	2	3	1	1	3	1	3	2	3	3	2	VA in 44.5%–AVB in 22.2%–LV dysfunction in 33.3%
AF (0 = no, 1 = yes)	1	1	1	0	0	0	0	0	0	1	0	0	0	1	0	0	0	1	7 (38.8)
VT/VF (0 = no, 1 = yes)	0	1	1	1	1	1	1	0	1	0	1	0	1	1	1	0	1	0	11 (61.1%)
ICD (0 = no, 1 = yes)	0	1	1	0	1	1	1	1	1	1	1	0	1	1	1	0	1	0	12 (66.6%)
ICD Therapy	/	0	1	/	0	1	1	0	1	0	1	/	1	1	0	0	1	/	8/12 (66.6)

CG: cardiogenetic samples; LMNA: Lamin A/C gene; LVEDD: left ventricular end-diastolic diameter; LVEDDi: left ventricular end-diastolic diameter index; EF: ejection fraction; CMR: cardiovascular magnetic resonance; LVEDV: left ventricular end-diastolic volume; LVEDVi: left ventricular end-diastolic volume index; cQT: corrected QT interval; LA: left atrium; RV: right ventricle; IVS: intraventricular septum; VA: ventricular delay; LBBB: left bundle branch block; AVB: atrioventricular block; AV: atrioventricular delay; IV: intraventricular delay; arrhythmias; AF: atrial fibrillation; VT/VF: ventricular tachycardia/ventricular fibrillation; ICD: implantable cardioverter–defibrillator.

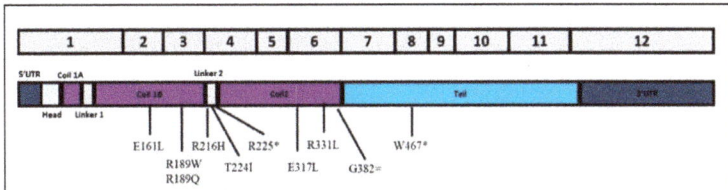

Figure 1. Schematic representation of lamin A transcript and localization of exonic variants identified in this study. * stands for nonsense mutations while = stands for synonymous mutations.

In eight patients (CG02, CG03, CG05, CG06, CG07, CG09, CG10, and CG11), whose clinical onset was characterized by ventricular arrhythmias, ICD was implanted as secondary prevention before diagnosis of lamin cardiomyopathy, as well as in another patient (CG12) that presented as the first phenotypic sign a severe reduction of the LVEF (20%); ICD was implanted as primary prevention before diagnosis of the LMNA variant.

Two patients (CG8A and CG14A) had a moderate LV dysfunction (LVEF 44% and 45%) and underwent ICD implantation after diagnosis of laminopathy because they both met the criteria for ICD implantation (as reported in the discussion, the European Guidelines recommend ICD implantation in lamin DCM if two of the following risk factors are present: male sex, non-sustained VT, non-missense variant, and LVEF < 45%):

- CG08 three factors: male sex, non-missense variant, LVEF 44%
- CG14A two factors: male sex, LVEF 45%

One patient (CG13) had already undergone PMK implantation for AVB, and once diagnosis of LMNA variant was made, an upgrade to ICD was performed (male sex, evidence of VA at PMK interrogation). A mean follow-up of 31.5 months was achieved, during which seven (38.8%) patients experienced AF; two patients (14%) developed new AVB. Eleven (61.1%) patients experienced VA. At ICD interrogation, 8 of 12 patients (66.6%) received an appropriate ICD therapy (shock in 62.5%) (Table 3).

One patient (CG12) received heart transplantation for end-stage heart failure. Regarding the remaining five patients without a DCM clinical phenotype, all clinical and instrumental assessments were normal except for the presence of LA dilatation in two of them (two young brothers, IV7 and IV9, belonging to Family 14, with a left atrium volume of, respectively, 36.1 and 39.6 mL/m^2).

3.2. In Vitro Characterization of Two Novel LMNA Variants

One patient belonging to Family 6 (III-2) and two brothers belonging to Family 14 (IV-7 and IV-9) underwent dermal biopsy in order to obtain in vitro fibroblasts (HDFs) (Figure 2). The missense R189Q variant of unknown significance (VUS) segregates in the daughter (IV-1) but not in the sibling (III-3 and III-4) of Family 6 (Figure 2A). In Family 14 (Figure 2B), the missense E317K is classified on ClinVar as likely pathogenic for DCM and reported in an Italian family with DCM and atrioventricular block [4].

Both lamin A/C and prelamin expression have been investigated, comparing them to healthy controls (WT). Lamin A/C localization, mainly situated at the nuclear peripheric rim, was comparable between WT and DCM-derived HDFs (99.8% positive cells), after immunofluorescence staining (Figure 3A). About 4.3% of WT nuclei were positive for prelamin A, as well as the IV-7 and IV-9 nuclei (5% and 4.98%, respectively), while III-2 nuclei (Family 6) were 12.2%. In these cells, a more punctate localization pattern relative to prelamin A was also revealed. These intra-nuclear aggregates differ significantly in size and number between cells within the same culture, and they are distributed next to a typical nuclear rim (Figure 3A, III-2). The total number of abnormal nuclei, which includes herniations, honeycomb-structures, and donut-like nuclei was found to be the most discriminating parameter between patient and control cells. In fact, 6% of IV-7, 7.7% of IV-9, and 6.68% of III-2 nuclei showed an altered shape with nuclear invaginations and blebs, considered typical markers associated with LMNA variants (Figure 3A,B). Results have evidenced statistically significant differences in circularity, roundness, and nuclear elongation (Figure 3C, * $p < 0.05$). The percentage of DCM irregular nuclei strongly increases compared to WT cells, in which these alterations are present only in 1%, at the same age and number of passages (p3) (Figure 3B,C).

Successively, transcript and protein expression have been evaluated (Figure 3D), comparing quantitatively lamin A and C in DCMs with respect to WTs. In all patients, both lamin isoforms were decreased compared to WT in a statistically significant manner, except for the IV-7 patient, in whom lamin A expression slightly increased (Figure 3D). Protein quantification performed by Western blot confirmed a marked reduction of both lamin A and C isoforms (Figure 3E,F), except in IV-7, as expected, who did not show any significant protein reduction (Figure 3E).

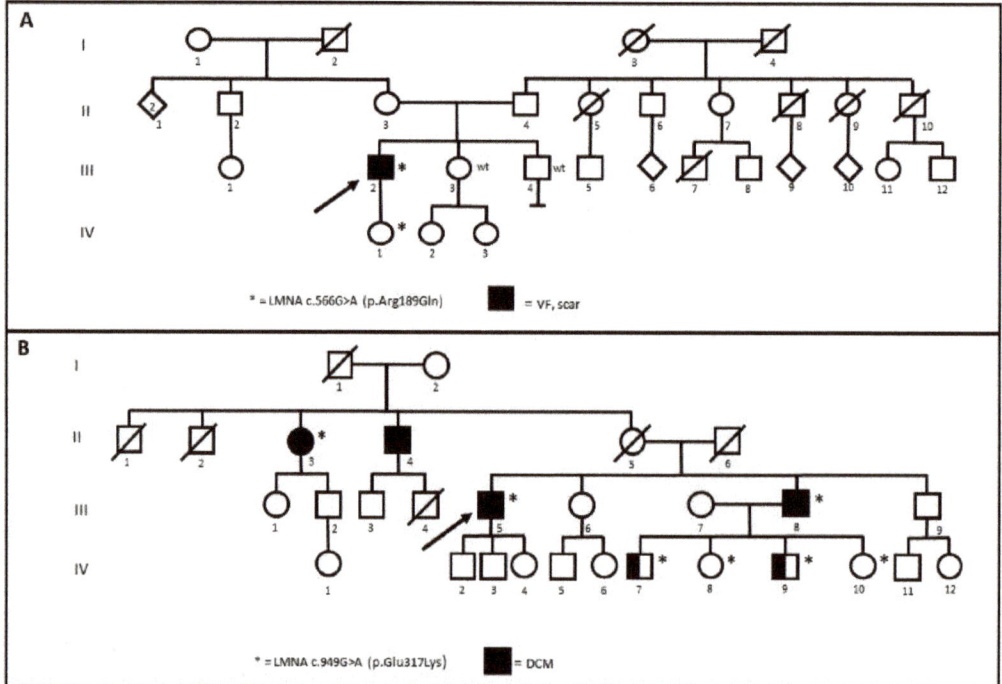

Figure 2. (**A**) Segregation of R189Q in Family 6. (**B**) Segregation of E317K in Family 14. Arrows indicate the proband. Wt: wild type. * stands for positive patients to Lamin A/C gene (LMNA) variants.

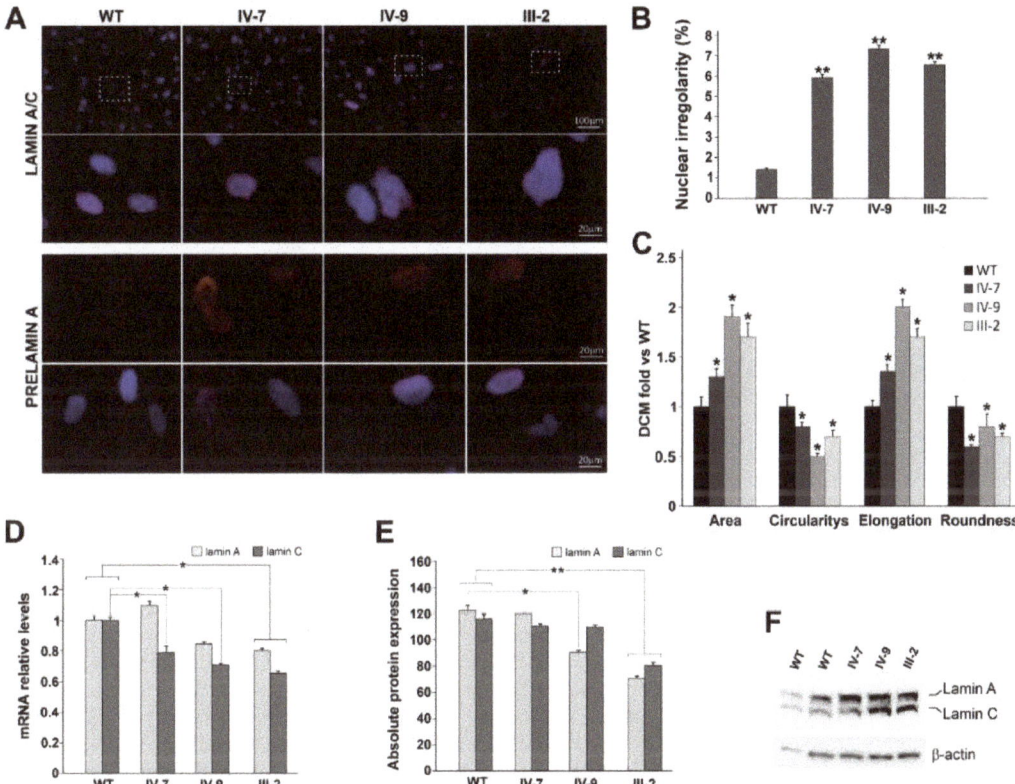

Figure 3. (**A**) Representative immunolabeling for lamin A/C (red) and Prelamin A (red) of WT and DCM HDFs (IV-7, IV-9, and III-2). Nuclei are counterstained with Hoechst 33,342 (blue). Scale bar 20 µm, 100 µm. (**B**) Percentage of WT and DCM cells with abnormal nuclear irregularities revealed in HDFs patients. Results represent three independent experiments with significant differences between WT and DCM HDFs (** $p < 0.01$). (**C**) Bar graphs represent the four parameters relative to nuclear shape (area; circularity; elongation; roundness); they are reported as mean values ± SD (fold DCM vs. WT) of three independent experiments. Significant differences are denoted by the p-value (Student's two-tailed t-test; * $p < 0.05$. (**D**) RT-qPCR of lamin A and C transcripts in WT and DCM HDFs; GAPDH was used as reference gene. Data are from three independent experiments and represented as mean ± SD (* $p < 0.05$). (**E**) Densitometric analysis of Western blot performed on WT and DCM HDFs, showing the intensity of the band corresponding to lamin A and C normalized versus β-actin levels. WT densitometric value is the average between two different controls (* $p < 0.05$; ** $p < 0.01$). Data are presented as mean ± SD. (**F**) Representative Western blot of lamin A and C; β-actin is used as housekeeping gene.

4. Discussion

LMNA-related DCMs have a more aggressive clinical course compared to other forms of dilated cardiomyopathies with higher rates of potentially fatal arrhythmias and end-stage heart failure [25]. The prevalence of LMNA mutations in familial DCM is about 5–10% [26]; however, only in 30–35% of familial cases, a Mendelian inheritance has been evidenced, suggesting a prevalent complex multi-variant or oligogenic basis of inheritance [27]. Moreover, a significant clinical heterogeneity has been reported within the same family in terms of onset, severity, and progression of the disease [28]. Both the genetic and phenotypic heterogeneities together with variable penetrance of LMNA variants make the pathogenic classification of the variants difficult.

LMNA variants occur in the head and rod domains, which comprise more than half of lamin A and two thirds of lamin C, but rarely in the tail domain [28]. The clinical heterogeneity observed in LMNA-DCM might be also explained by the different functional consequences of the variants. Most carriers exhibit an age-dependent penetrance: 7% under the age of 20 years to 100% above the age of 60 years [17].

Actually, a targeted therapy is not available for the early treatment of LMNA associated cardiac disease. However, the knowledge of the genotype of DCM patients allows a better prevention with ICD because of the high risk of SCD associated with LMNA variants.

The introduction of the NGS method in the daily practice of molecular diagnosis laboratories has allowed considerably reducing response times. The possibility to identify genetic variations in DCM patients allows early diagnosis before clinical manifestation, prognosis, genetic counselling, and preventive management of heterozygous subjects and their relatives.

In our cohort of patients with DCM, LMNA variants are present in about 19.5%. This finding is not in line with previous reports describing a 5–8% prevalence [29], probably because all patients come from a clinical center specialized in arrhythmology. Affected individuals frequently suffer from a progressive conduction system disease such as atrioventricular block, bradyarrhythmias, and tachyarrhythmias and have a high chance of developing thromboembolic disorder. It has been shown that men have a worse prognosis than women [30]; however, in our study, we have only three symptomatic female patients vs. 15 male patients, and we cannot draw any conclusions about this. Three variants described in our cohort belong to Class V, seven to Class IV, and one to Class III. Interestingly, the variant E317K was reported in Gnomad with only one allele count (frequency 3.19e-5), while in our study, it is present in six proband, allowing us to hypothesize a founder effect in the Italian population, as already reported for R331Q, a founder variant in autosomal dominant cardiac laminopathy with late-onset and mild cardiac phenotypes [31]. A specific study of haplotypes associated with this variant is necessary to confirm our hypothesis. Segregation analysis performed within each family lets us identify five members in the presymptomatic stage.

In total, 11 LMNA variants were identified in 15 families, and, as expected, phenotype-positive patients showed a complex cardiac phenotype ranging from a predominantly structural heart disease to a highly arrhythmic profile in an apparently normal heart. VA were the first relief in 44.5% of patients. This finding is of particular interest since VA generally do not appear as first clinical manifestation [32], with prevalence of any and all forms of sustained VA increasing from presentation to last follow-up [33].

Moreover, 62.5% of patients who experienced VT/VF as a first manifestation had a LVEF ≥50%. At follow-up, VA occurred in up to 61.1% of patients, and 66.6% of ICD-implanted patients received appropriate ICD therapy.

These data highlight once again the highly arrhythmic burden of LMNA-related DCM and the limits of systolic function in risk stratification, emphasizing instead the importance of a gene-based diagnosis. Systolic function evaluation is an important prognostic factor in DCM, but our data suggest its marginal role in predicting the risk of VA in patients with LMNA variants. Probably the early appearance of interstitial fibrosis together with ion channels anomalies [34] could represent the cause of ventricular arrhythmias even before systolic dysfunction occurs. In fact, as already recognized [35], the presence of a scar at CMR, generally located in the IVS, is extremely frequent in asymptomatic patients, and it represents a potential trigger of VA, explaining why VA often represents the first clinical manifestation in asymptomatic patients. In our study, MRI evidenced a scar in 87.5% of the patients who experienced VA. Moreover, EF represents only one of the four independent risk factors for malignant VA identified in lamin DCM: male sex, non-sustained VT, non-missense variant, and LVEF < 45% [32]. According to the actual European Guidelines for the management of patients with ventricular arrhythmias and the prevention of sudden cardiac death, ICD implantation in patient carriers of lamin variants should be considered when two of the above mentioned criteria are met [36]. The genetic analyses would be useful not only for diagnosing the laminopathy, but also for stratifying the prognosis of carriers [37].

Patients with LMNA-related DCM frequently face supraventricular arrhythmias including atrial fibrillation, atrial flutter, and focal atrial tachycardia, as expression of atrial disease [38]. In our study, the prevalence of supraventricular arrhythmias was 38.8% at follow-up, in line with other studies [33,39]. A common relief in our population was left atrial enlargement, found in 83.3% of symptomatic patients. Left atrial size is a well-known predisposal factor for the occurrence of supraventricular arrhythmias, especially AF [40–42], commonly proposed as a barometer of diastolic burden and a predictor of common cardiovascular outcomes and cardiovascular death [43,44]. In our study, left atrial enlargement was the only abnormal finding evidenced in the two older male patients, aged 22 and 27 years, of the five total genotype positive asymptomatic patients. A third patient, female biological sex aged 26 years, showed an upper limit LA volume. Although this evidence comes from a low number of patients, we could speculate about atrial enlargement as an early marker of the disease in LMNA cardiomyopathies, rather than a mere consequence of pressure and/or volume overload due to LV dysfunction and worse LV compliance. The LA enlargement due to a "primitive LMNA induced atrial myopathy", if confirmed in further studies, could represent an important relief to look for in genotype-positive phenotype-negative subjects, as initial sign of structural heart disease. Moreover, defining molecular and cellular mechanism causing the "primitive LMNA induced atrial myopathy" could lead to identify novel pathogenic mechanisms involved in supraventricular arrhythmias' occurrence.

Successively, lamin expression and distribution were evaluated in vitro on HDFs carrying two novel LMNA variants: R189Q and E317K. Moreover, nuclear abnormalities and irregularities in lamin staining were assessed in order to correlate them to variant nature and disease phenotype [45–49]. The increased percentage of abnormal nuclei, irrespective of the type of nuclear malformation, is the most discriminating parameter between normal and lamin-defective cells [50], correlating with nuclear architecture instability [51]. Lamins are components of the nuclear lamina providing mechanical stability to the nucleus [52–57]. HDFs carrying R189Q displayed an abnormal prelamin accumulation, which usually correlates with senescent cells and premature aging. Accumulated prelamin A causes the captures of the transcription factor Sp1, resulting in altered extracellular matrix gene expression [58]. Nuclear dysmorphisms and nuclear envelope disorganization appear as a hallmark of human cultured laminopathic cells, independently of the associated clinical presentation [49,59,60].

Additionally, the transcription levels of both Lamin A and Lamin C have been evaluated. They are usually incorporated in the nuclear lamina in equivalent amounts and play distinct functions: any expression ratio variations may be due to altered splicing or mRNA stability [52].

In all patients, lamin C expression is statistically significantly reduced if compared to WT ones. In the III-2 patient, lamin A was also significantly reduced. Overall, lamin A/C ratio is modified from 1:1 value, especially in IV-7, in whom lamin A expression increased with respect to the younger brother. This unbalance, due to an aberrant splicing process, may lead to altered interaction with other important structural proteins and transcription factors, as well as altered chromatin interaction [61]. These data are confirmed at protein level in III-2 and IV-9 patients, expressing lower quantities of both protein isoforms, as evidenced by densitometric analysis of Western blot, suggesting a possible defective mechanotransduction and an enhanced nuclear fragility.

Importantly, the different behavior between two brothers (IV-7 and IV-9) in lamin expression can explain the worse DCM phenotype evidenced in the youngest one. These data confirm the key role played by lamin in conferring a greater susceptibility to physical stress, especially in tissues exposed to mechanical strain, such as cardiac muscle [62].

Supplementary Materials: The following are available online at https://www.mdpi.com/article/10.3390/jcm10215075/s1, Table S1: Genes sequenced for SCD.

Author Contributions: Conceptualization, V.F., J.C., F.S. and R.M.; methodology, V.F., J.C., P.S., M.M. and C.D.M.; validation, F.S., G.N., L.C., F.F. and R.M.; formal analysis, F.R., S.M., G.P., F.D.L. and A.M.; data curation, J.C. and V.F.; writing—original draft preparation, J.C., V.F., M.M. and P.S.; writing—review and editing, F.S. and R.M.; supervision, F.S., R.M., G.N. and L.C.; project administration, F.S. and R.M. All authors have read and agreed to the published version of the manuscript.

Funding: This research received no external funding.

Institutional Review Board Statement: The study was conducted according to the guidelines of the Declaration of Helsinki and approved by Committees on Health Research Ethics of Tor Vergata Hospital n.2932/2017.

Informed Consent Statement: Informed consent was obtained from all subjects involved in the study.

Data Availability Statement: Variant submitted to ClinVar, Submission ID: SUB9594435.

Acknowledgments: Authors thank clinicians and patients for their collaboration.

Conflicts of Interest: The authors declare no conflict of interest.

References

1. Richardson, P.; McKenna, W.; Bristow, M.; Maisch, B.; Mautner, B.; O'Connell, J.; Olsenet, E.; Thiene, G.; Goodwin, J.; Gyarfas, I.; et al. Report of the 1995 World Health Organ-ization/International Society and Federation of Cardiology Task Force on the Definition and Classification of cardio-myopathies. *Circulation* **1996**, *93*, 841–842.
2. Watkins, H.; Ashrafian, H.; Redwood, C. Inherited cardiomyopathies. *N. Engl. J. Med.* **2011**, *364*, 1643–1656. [CrossRef]
3. Hershberger, R.E.; Morales, A. LMNA-Related Dilated Cardiomyopathy. In *GeneReviews®*; University of Washington: Seattle, WA, USA, 1993.
4. Arbustini, E.; Pilotto, A.; Repetto, A.; Grasso, M.; Negri, A.; Diegoli, M.; Campana, C.; Scelsi, L.; Baldini, E.; Gavazzi, A.; et al. Autosomal dominant dilated cardiomyopathy with atrioventricular block: A lamin A/C defect-related disease. *J. Am. Coll. Cardiol.* **2002**, *39*, 981–990. [CrossRef]
5. Fawcett, D.W. On the occurrence of a fibrous lamina on the inner aspect of the nuclear envelope in certain cells of vertebrates. *Am. J. Anat.* **1966**, *119*, 129–145. [CrossRef]
6. Bouhouche, A.; Benomar, A.; Birouk, N.; Mularoni, A.; Meggouh, F.; Tassin, J.; Grid, D.; Vandenberghe, A.; Yahyaoui, M.; Chkili, T.; et al. A Locus for an Axonal Form of Autosomal Recessive Charcot-Marie-Tooth Disease Maps to Chromosome 1q21.2-q21.3. *Am. J. Hum. Genet.* **1999**, *65*, 722–727. [CrossRef]
7. Lin, F.; Worman, H. Structural organization of the human gene encoding nuclear lamin A and nuclear lamin C. *J. Biol. Chem.* **1993**, *268*, 16321–16326. [CrossRef]
8. Gerbino, A.; Procino, G.; Svelto, M.; Carmosino, M. Role of Lamin A/C Gene Mutations in the Signaling Defects Leading to Cardiomyopathies. *Front. Physiol.* **2018**, *9*, 1356. [CrossRef]
9. Swift, J.; Discher, D.E. The nuclear lamina is mechano-responsive to ECM elasticity in mature tissue. *J. Cell Sci.* **2014**, *127*, 3005–3015. [CrossRef]
10. Gruenbaum, Y.; Foisner, R. Lamins: Nuclear intermediate filament proteins with fundamental functions in nuclear mechanics and genome regulation. *Annu. Rev. Biochem.* **2015**, *84*, 131–164. [CrossRef]
11. Rankin, J.; Ellard, S. The laminopathies: A clinical review. *Clin. Genet.* **2006**, *70*, 261–274. [CrossRef]
12. D'Apice, M.R.; De Dominicis, A.; Murdocca, M.; Amati, F.; Botta, A.; Sangiuolo, F.; Lattanzi, G.; Federici, M.; Novelli, G. Cutaneous and metabolic defects associated with nuclear abnormalities in a transgenic mouse model expressing R527H lamin A mutation causing mandibuloacral dysplasia type A (MADA) syndrome. *Acta Myol.* **2020**, *39*, 320–335.
13. Brodt, C.; Siegfried, J.D.; Hofmeyer, M.; Martel, J.; Rampersaud, E.; Li, D.; Morales, A.; Hershberger, R.E. Temporal Relationship of Conduction System Disease and Ventricular Dysfunction in LMNA Cardiomyopathy. *J. Card. Fail.* **2013**, *19*, 233–239. [CrossRef]
14. Taylor, M.D.; Towbin, J.A. The Significant Arrhythmia and Cardiomyopathy Burden of Lamin A/C Mutations. *J. Am. Coll. Cardiol.* **2016**, *68*, 2308–2310. [CrossRef]
15. Pasotti, M.; Klersy, C.; Pilotto, A.; Marziliano, N.; Rapezzi, C.; Serio, A.; Mannarino, S.; Gambarin, F.I.; Favalli, V.; Grasso, M.; et al. Long-Term Outcome and Risk Stratification in Dilated Cardiolaminopathies. *J. Am. Coll. Cardiol.* **2008**, *52*, 1250–1260. [CrossRef]
16. Fatkin, D.; MacRae, C.; Sasaki, T.; Wolff, M.R.; Porcu, M.; Frenneaux, M.; Atherton, J.; Vidaillet, H.J., Jr.; Spudich, S.; De Girolami, U.; et al. Missense mutations in the rod domain of the lamin A/C gene as causes of dilated cardiomyopathy and conduction-system disease. *N. Engl. J. Med.* **1999**, *341*, 1715–1724. [CrossRef]
17. Taylor, M.R.; Fain, P.R.; Sinagra, G.; Robinson, M.L.; Robertson, A.D.; Carniel, E.; Di Lenarda, A.; Bohlmeyer, T.J.; A Ferguson, D.; Brodsky, G.L.; et al. Natural history of dilated cardiomyopathy due to lamin A/C gene mutations. *J. Am. Coll. Cardiol.* **2003**, *41*, 771–780. [CrossRef]
18. Charron, P.; Arbustini, E.; Bonne, G. What Should the Cardiologist know about Lamin Disease? *Arrhythmia Electrophysiol. Rev.* **2012**, *1*, 22–28. [CrossRef]

19. Mestroni, L.; Maisch, B.; McKenna, W.J.; Schwartz, K.; Charron, P.; Rocco, C.; Tesson, F.; Richter, A.; Wilke, A.; Komajda, M. Guidelines for the study of familial dilated cardiomyopathies. Collaborative Research Group of the European Human and Capital Mobility Project on Familial Dilated Cardiomyopathy. *Eur. Heart J.* **1999**, *20*, 93–102. [CrossRef]
20. Kramer, C.M.; Barkhausen, J.; Bucciarelli-Ducci, C.; Flamm, S.D.; Kim, J.R.; Nagel, E. Standardized cardiovascular magnetic resonance imaging (CMR) protocols: 2020 update. *J. Cardiovasc. Magn. Reson.* **2020**, *22*, 17. [CrossRef]
21. Schulz-Menger, J.; Bluemke, D.A.; Bremerich, J.; Flamm, S.D.; Fogel, M.A.; Friedrich, M.G.; Kim, R.J.; von Knobelsdorff-Brenkenhoff, F.; Kramer, C.M.; Pennell, D.J.; et al. Standardized image in-terpretation and post processing in cardiovascular magnetic resonance: Society for Cardiovascular Magnetic Resonance (SCMR) Board of Trustees Task Force on Standardized Post Processing. *J. Cardiovasc. Magn. Reson.* **2013**, *1*, 15–35.
22. Kawel-Boehm, N.; Maceira, A.; Valsangiacomo-Buechel, E.R.; Vogel-Claussen, J.; Turkbey, E.B.; Williams, R.; Plein, S.; Tee, M.; Eng, J.; Bluemke, A.D. Normal values for cardiovascular magnetic resonance in adults and children. *J. Cardiovasc. Magn. Reson.* **2015**, *17*, 29. [CrossRef]
23. Spitalieri, P.; Talarico, R.V.; Caioli, S.; Murdocca, M.; Serafino, A.; Girasole, M.; Dinarelli, S.; Longo, G.; Pucci, S.; Botta, A.; et al. Modelling the pathogenesis of Myotonic Dystrophy type 1 cardiac phenotype through human iPSC-derived cardiomyocytes. *J. Mol. Cell Cardiol.* **2018**, *118*, 95–109. [CrossRef]
24. Richards, S.; Aziz, N.; Bale, S.; Bick, D.; Das, S.; Gastrier-Foster, J.; Grody, W.W.; Hedge, M.; Lyon, E.; Spector, E.; et al. Standards and guidelines for the interpretation of sequence variants: A joint consensus recommendation of the American College of Medical Genetics and Genomics and the Association for Molecular Pathology. *Genet. Med.* **2015**, *17*, 405–424. [CrossRef]
25. van Berlo, J.H.; de Voogt, W.G.; van der Kooi, A.J.; van Tintelen, J.P.; Bonne, G.; Ben Yaou, R.; Duboc, D.; Rossenbacher, T.; Heidbüchel, H.; de Visser, M.; et al. Meta-analysis of clinical characteristics of 299 carriers of LMNA gene mutations: Do lamin A/C mutations portend a high risk of sudden death? *J. Mol. Med.* **2005**, *83*, 79–83. [CrossRef]
26. Perrot, A.; Hussein, S.; Ruppert, V.; Schmidt, H.H.J.; Wehnert, M.S.; Duong, N.T.; Posch, M.G.; Panek, A.; Dietz, R.; Kindermann, I.; et al. Identification of mutational hot spots in LMNA encoding lamin A/C in patients with familial dilated cardiomyopathy. *Basic Res. Cardiol.* **2009**, *104*, 90–99. [CrossRef]
27. Hershberger, R.E.; Hedges, D.J.; Morales, A. Dilated cardiomyopathy: The complexity of a diverse genetic architecture. *Nat. Rev. Cardiol.* **2013**, *10*, 531–547. [CrossRef]
28. Zahr, H.C.; Jaalouk, D.E. Exploring the Crosstalk between LMNA and Splicing Machinery Gene Mutations in Dilated Cardiomyopathy. *Front. Genet.* **2018**, *9*, 231. [CrossRef]
29. Jacoby, D.; McKenna, W.J. Genetics of inherited cardiomyopathy. *Eur. Hear. J.* **2011**, *33*, 296–304. [CrossRef]
30. van Rijsingen, I.A.; Nannenberg, E.A.; Arbustini, E.; Elliot, P.M.; Mogensen, J.; Hermans-van Ast, J.F.; van der Kooi, A.J.; van Tintelen, J.P.; van den Berg, M.P.; Grasso, M.; et al. Gender-specific dif-ferences in major cardiac events and mortality in lamin A/C mutation carriers. *Eur. J. Heart. Fail.* **2013**, *15*, 376–384. [CrossRef]
31. Hoorntje, E.T.; Bollen, I.A.; Barge-Schaapveld, D.Q.; van Tienen, F.H.; te Meerman, G.J.; Jansweijer, J.A.; van Essen, A.J.; Volders, P.G.; Constantinescu, A.A.; van den Akker, P.C.; et al. LMNA-related cardiac disease: Late onset with a variable and mild phenotype in a large cohort of patients with the LMNA p.(Arg331Gln) founder mutation. *Circ. Cardiovasc. Genet.* **2017**, *10*, e001631. [CrossRef]
32. van Rijsingen, I.A.; Arbustini, E.; Elliott, P.M.; Mogensen, J.; Hermans-van Ast, J.F.; van der Kooi, A.J.; van Tintelen, J.P.; van den Berg, M.P.; Pilotto, A.; Pasotti, M.; et al. Risk factors for malignant ventricular arrhythmias in lamin a/c mutation carriers a European cohort study. *J. Am. Coll. Cardiol.* **2012**, *59*, 493–500. [CrossRef]
33. Kumar, S.; Baldinger, S.H.; Gandjbakhch, E.; Maury, P.; Sellal, J.-M.; Androulakis, A.F.; Waintraub, X.; Charron, P.; Rollin, A.; Richard, P.; et al. Long-Term Arrhythmic and Nonarrhythmic Outcomes of Lamin A/C Mutation Carriers. *J. Am. Coll. Cardiol.* **2016**, *68*, 2299–2307. [CrossRef]
34. El-Battrawy, I.; Zhao, Z.; Lan, H.; Li, X.; Yücel, G.; Lang, S.; Sattler, K.; Schünemann, J.-D.; Zimmermann, W.-H.; Cyganek, L.; et al. Ion Channel Dysfunctions in Dilated Cardiomyopathy in Limb-Girdle Muscular Dystrophy. *Circ. Genom. Precis. Med.* **2018**, *11*, e001893. [CrossRef]
35. Holmström, M.; Kivistö, S.; Heliö, T.; Jurkko, R.; Kaartinen, M.; Antila, M.; Reissell, E.; Kuusisto, J.; Kärkkäinen, S.; Peuhkurinen, K.; et al. Late gadolinium enhanced cardiovascular magnetic resonance of lamin A/C gene mutation related dilated cardiomyopathy. *J. Cardiovasc. Magn. Reson.* **2011**, *13*, 30. [CrossRef]
36. Priori, S.G.; Blomström-Lundqvist, C.; Mazzanti, A.; Blom, N.; Borggrefe, M.; Camm, J.; Elliott, P.M.; Fitzsimons, D.; Hatala, R.; Hindricks, G.; et al. 2015 ESC Guidelines for the management of patients with ventricular arrhythmias and the prevention of sudden cardiac death: The Task Force for the Management of Patients with Ventricular Arrhythmias and the Prevention of Sudden Cardiac Death of the European Society of Cardiology (ESC) Endorsed by: Association for European Paediatric and Congenital Cardiology (AEPC). *Eur. Heart J.* **2015**, *36*, 2793–2867.
37. Fujino, N.; Hayashi, K.; Sakata, K.; Nomura, A.; Kawashiri, M.-A. Phenotype and Prognosis of the Lamin A/C Gene (LMNA) Mutation Carriers in Japan. *Circ. J.* **2018**, *82*, 2699–2700. [CrossRef]
38. Peretto, G.; Sala, S.; Benedetti, S.; Di Resta, C.; Gigli, L.; Ferrari, M.; Della Bella, P. Updated clinical overview on cardiac laminopathies: An electrical and mechanical disease. *Nucleus* **2018**, *9*, 380–391. [CrossRef]

39. Hasselberg, N.E.; Haland, T.F.; Saberniak, J.; Brekke, P.; Berge, K.E.; Leren, T.P.; Edvardsen, T.; Haugaa, K. Lamin A/C cardiomyopathy: Young onset, high penetrance, and frequent need for heart transplantation. *Eur. Heart J.* **2018**, *39*, 853–860. [CrossRef]
40. Mont, L.; Tamborero, D.; Elosua, R.; Molina, I.; Coll-Vinent, B.; Sitges, M.; Vidal, B.; Scalise, A.; Tejeira, A.; Berruezo, A.; et al. Physical activity, height, and left atrial size are independent risk factors for lone atrial fibrillation in middle-aged healthy individuals. *Europace* **2008**, *10*, 15–20. [CrossRef]
41. Thomas, L.; Abhayaratna, W.P. Left Atrial Reverse Remodeling: Mechanisms, Evaluation, and Clinical Significance. *JACC Cardiovasc. Imaging* **2017**, *10*, 65–77. [CrossRef]
42. Tsang, T.S.; Barnes, M.E.; Bailey, K.R.; Leibson, C.L.; Montgomery, S.C.; Takemoto, Y.; Diamond, P.M.; Marra, M.A.; Gersh, B.J.; Wiebers, D.O.; et al. Left atrial volume: Important risk marker of incident atrial fibrillation in 1,655 older men and women. *Mayo Clin. Proc.* **2001**, *76*, 467–475. [CrossRef]
43. Rossi, A.; Cicoira, M.; Zanolla, L.; Sandrini, R.; Golia, G.; Zardini, P.; Enriquez-Sarano, M. Determinants and prognostic value of left atrial volume in patients with dilated cardiomyopathy. *J. Am. Coll. Cardiol.* **2002**, *40*, 1425–1430. [CrossRef]
44. Tsang, T.S.; E Barnes, M.; Gersh, B.J.; Bailey, K.R.; Seward, J.B. Risks for atrial fibrillation and congestive heart failure in patients ≥65 years of age with abnormal left ventricular diastolic relaxation. *Am. J. Cardiol.* **2004**, *93*, 54–58. [CrossRef]
45. Novelli, G.; Muchir, A.; Sangiuolo, F.; Helbling-Leclerc, A.; D'Apice, M.R.; Massart, C.; Capon, F.; Sbraccia, P.; Federici, M.; Lauro, R.; et al. Mandibuloacral dysplasia is caused by a mutation in LMNA-encoding lamin A/C. *Am. J. Hum. Genet.* **2002**, *71*, 426–431. [CrossRef]
46. Vigouroux, C.; Auclair, M.; Dubosclard, E.; Pouchelet, M.; Capeau, J.; Courvalin, J.C.; Buendia, B. Nuclear envelope disorganization in fibroblasts from lipodystrophic patients with heterozygous R482Q/W mutations in the lamin A/C gene. *J. Cell Sci.* **2001**, *114*, 4459–4468. [CrossRef]
47. Fidzianska, A.; Bilinska, Z.T.; Tesson, F.; Wagner, T.; Walski, M.; Grzybowski, J.; Ruzyłło, W.; Hausmanowa-Petrusewicz, I. Obliteration of cardiomyocyte nuclear architecture in a patient with LMNA gene mutation. *J. Neurol. Sci.* **2008**, *271*, 91–96. [CrossRef]
48. Gupta, P.; Bilinska, Z.T.; Sylvius, N.; Boudreau, E.; Veinot, J.P.; Labib, S.; Bolongo, P.M.; Hamza, A.; Jackson, T.; Ploski, R.; et al. Genetic and ultrastructural studies in dilated cardiomyopathy patients: A large deletion in the lamin A/C gene is associated with cardiomyocyte nuclear envelope disruption. *Basic Res. Cardiol.* **2010**, *105*, 365–377. [CrossRef]
49. Muchir, A.; Medioni, J.; Laluc, M.; Massart, C.; Arimura, T.; Van Der Kooi, A.J.; Desguerre, I.; Mayer, M.; Ferrer, X.; Briault, S.; et al. Nuclear envelope alterations in fibroblasts from patients with muscular dystrophy, cardiomyopathy, and partial lipodystrophy carrying lamin A/C gene mutations. *Muscle Nerve* **2004**, *30*, 444–450. [CrossRef]
50. van Tienen, F.H.J.; Lindsey, P.J.; Kamps, M.A.F.; Krapels, I.P.; Ramaekers, F.C.S.; Brunner, H.G.; van den Wijngaard, A.; Broers, J.L.V. Assessment of fibroblast nuclear morphology aids interpretation of LMNA variants. *Eur. J. Hum. Genet.* **2019**, *27*, 389–399. [CrossRef]
51. Lee, J.; Termglinchan, V.; Diecke, S.; Itzhaki, I.; Lam, C.K.; Garg, P.; Lau, E.; Greenhaw, M.; Seeger, T.; Wu, H.; et al. Activation of PDGF pathway links LMNA mutation to dilated cardiomyopathy. *Nat. Cell Biol.* **2019**, *572*, 335–340. [CrossRef]
52. Burke, B.; Stewart, C.L. The nuclear lamins: Flexibility in function. *Nat. Rev. Mol. Cell Biol.* **2013**, *14*, 13–24. [CrossRef]
53. Zuela, N.; Bar, D.Z.; Gruenbaum, Y. Lamins in development, tissue maintenance and stress. *EMBO Rep.* **2012**, *13*, 1070–1078. [CrossRef] [PubMed]
54. Choi, J.C.; Worman, H.J. Nuclear Envelope Regulation of Signaling Cascades. *Adv. Exp. Med. Biol.* **2014**, *773*, 187–206. [CrossRef]
55. Kennedy, B.K.; Pennypacker, J.K. RB and Lamins in Cell Cycle Regulation and Aging. *Adv. Exp. Med. Biol.* **2014**, *773*, 127–142. [CrossRef]
56. Shimi, T.; Goldman, R.D. Nuclear Lamins and Oxidative Stress in Cell Proliferation and Longevity. *Adv. Exp. Med. Biol.* **2014**, *773*, 415–430. [CrossRef]
57. Isermann, P.; Lammerding, J. Nuclear Mechanics and Mechanotransduction in Health and Disease. *Curr. Biol.* **2013**, *23*, R1113–R1121. [CrossRef]
58. Ruiz de Eguino, G.; Infante, A.; Schlangen, K.; Aransay, A.M.; Fullaondo, A.; Soriano, M.; García-Verdugo, J.M.; Martín, A.G.; Rodríguez, C.I. Sp1 transcription factor interaction with accumulated prelamin a impairs adipose lineage differentiation in human mesenchymal stem cells: Essential role of sp1 in the integrity of lipid vesicles. *Stem Cells Transl. Med.* **2012**, *1*, 309–321. [CrossRef]
59. Goldman, R.D.; Shumaker, D.K.; Erdos, M.R.; Eriksson, M.; Goldman, A.E.; Gordon, L.B.; Gruenbaum, Y.; Khuon, S.; Mendez, M.; Varga, R.; et al. Accumulation of mutant lamin A causes progressive changes in nuclear architecture in Hutchinson–Gilford progeria syndrome. *Proc. Natl. Acad. Sci. USA* **2004**, *101*, 8963–8968. [CrossRef]
60. Caron, M.; Auclair, M.; Donadille, B.; Béréziat, V.; Guerci, B.; Laville, M.; Narbonne, H.; Bodemer, C.; Lascols, O.; Capeau, J.; et al. Human lipodystrophies linked to mutations in A-type lamins and to HIV protease inhibitor therapy are both associated with prelamin A accumulation, oxidative stress and premature cellular senescence. *Cell Death Differ.* **2007**, *14*, 1759–1767. [CrossRef]
61. Al-Saaidi, R.; Bross, P. Do lamin A and lamin C have unique roles? *Chromosoma* **2014**, *124*, 1–12. [CrossRef]
62. Magagnotti, C.; Bachi, A.; Zerbini, G.; Fattore, E.; Fermo, I.; Riba, M.; Previtali, S.C.; Ferrari, M.; Andolfo, A.; Benedetti, S. Protein profiling reveals energy metabolism and cytoskeletal protein alterations in LMNA mutation carriers. *Biochim. Biophys. Acta (BBA)-Mol. Basis Dis.* **2012**, *1822*, 970–979. [CrossRef] [PubMed]

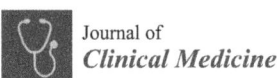

Article

Continuous Electrical Monitoring in Patients with Arrhythmic Myocarditis: Insights from a Referral Center

Giovanni Peretto [1,2,3,*], Patrizio Mazzone [1], Gabriele Paglino [1], Alessandra Marzi [1], Georgios Tsitsinakis [1], Stefania Rizzo [4], Cristina Basso [4], Paolo Della Bella [1] and Simone Sala [1,2]

1. Department of Cardiac Electrophysiology and Arrhythmology, IRCCS San Raffaele Scientific Institute, 20132 Milan, Italy; mazzone.patrizio@hsr.it (P.M.); paglino.grabriele@hsr.it (G.P.); marzi.alessandra@hsr.it (A.M.); gio.tsitsi@yahoo.gr (G.T.); dellabella.paolo@hsr.it (P.D.B.); sala.simone@hsr.it (S.S.)
2. Myocarditis Disease Unit, IRCCS San Raffaele Scientific Institute, 20132 Milan, Italy
3. School of Medicine, San Raffaele Vita-Salute University, 20132 Milan, Italy
4. Department of Cardiac Thoracic Vascular Sciences and Public Health, Cardiovascular Pathology, Padua University, 35128 Padua, Italy; s.rizzo@unipd.it (S.R.); cristina.basso@unipd.it (C.B.)
* Correspondence: peretto.giovanni@hsr.it; Tel./Fax: +39-02-2643-7484-7326

Citation: Peretto, G.; Mazzone, P.; Paglino, G.; Marzi, A.; Tsitsinakis, G.; Rizzo, S.; Basso, C.; Della Bella, P.; Sala, S. Continuous Electrical Monitoring in Patients with Arrhythmic Myocarditis: Insights from a Referral Center. *J. Clin. Med.* **2021**, *10*, 5142. https://doi.org/10.3390/jcm10215142

Academic Editor: Michael Henein

Received: 28 September 2021
Accepted: 29 October 2021
Published: 1 November 2021

Publisher's Note: MDPI stays neutral with regard to jurisdictional claims in published maps and institutional affiliations.

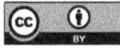

Copyright: © 2021 by the authors. Licensee MDPI, Basel, Switzerland. This article is an open access article distributed under the terms and conditions of the Creative Commons Attribution (CC BY) license (https://creativecommons.org/licenses/by/4.0/).

Abstract: Background. The incidence and burden of arrhythmias in myocarditis are under-reported. Objective. We aimed to assess the diagnostic yield and clinical impact of continuous arrhythmia monitoring (CAM) in patients with arrhythmic myocarditis. Methods. We enrolled consecutive adult patients (n = 104; 71% males, age 47 ± 11 year, mean LVEF 50 ± 13%) with biopsy-proven active myocarditis and de novo ventricular arrhythmias (VAs). All patients underwent prospective monitoring by both sequential 24-h Holter ECGs and CAM, including either ICD (n = 62; 60%) or loop recorder (n = 42; 40%). Results. By 3.7 ± 1.6 year follow up, 45 patients (43%) had VT, 67 (64%) NSVT and 102 (98%) premature ventricular complexes (PVC). As compared to the Holter ECG (average 9.5 exams per patient), CAM identified more patients with VA (VT: 45 vs. 4; NSVT: 64 vs. 45; both p < 0.001), more VA episodes (VT: 100 vs. 4%; NSVT: 91 vs. 12%) and earlier NSVT timing (median 6 vs. 24 months, p < 0.001). The extensive ICD implantation strategy was proven beneficial in 80% of the population. Histological signs of chronically active myocarditis (n = 73, 70%) and anteroseptal late gadolinium enhancement (n = 26, 25%) were significantly associated with the occurrence of VTs during follow up, even in the primary prevention subgroup. Conclusion. In patients with arrhythmic myocarditis, CAM allowed accurate arrhythmia detection and showed a considerable clinical impact.

Keywords: myocarditis; arrhythmias; telemonitoring; implantable cardioverter defibrillator; implantable loop recorder; Holter ECG

1. Introduction

Continuous arrhythmia monitoring (CAM) via implantable devices represents the gold standard for the detection of arrhythmias under many medical conditions [1,2]. In fact, in contrast to non-continuous monitoring by either Holter ECGs or short-term external devices [3], CAM allows the continuous and potentially life-long evaluation of cardiac electrical activity. In myocarditis, CAM may be useful to fill in relevant knowledge gaps on the incidence, type and burden of arrhythmias [4,5]. This is clinically important since ventricular arrhythmias (VAs) and bradyarrhythmias (BAs) constitute life-threatening complications of myocarditis [6,7]. Furthermore, the incidence of atrial fibrillation (AF) and other supraventricular arrhythmias (SVAs) is unknown in this setting. To date, no studies have investigated the benefits of CAM application in patients with myocarditis. In fact, indications for implantable cardioverter defibrillators (ICDs) are restricted in this population [5,6] and there is currently no experience about the use of implantable loop recorders (ILRs) as long-term monitoring devices. Because of the episodic nature of arrhythmias, we hypothesized that, even in the myocarditis population, CAM had a superior diagnostic yield compared to even regularly repeated Holter ECGs. In addition, we aimed to assess the appropriateness of the ICD implantation strategy in patients presenting with clinically defined acute myocarditis but heterogeneous histopathological findings.

2. Methods

2.1. Study Design

This was a single-center observational study with a prospective follow up reflecting the experience of a referral center. This study was in compliance with the Declaration of Helsinki and underwent Institutional Review Board approval. The study flowchart is presented in Figure 1. Between January 2013 and January 2019, consecutive patients with arrhythmic myocarditis were enrolled. The following inclusion criteria were applied: (1) age $\geq$ 18 year; (2) EMB-proven diagnosis of active myocarditis [5]; (3) evidence of previously unknown (or de novo) arrhythmias at index hospitalization; and (4) a CAM strategy started within 30 days from myocarditis diagnosis.

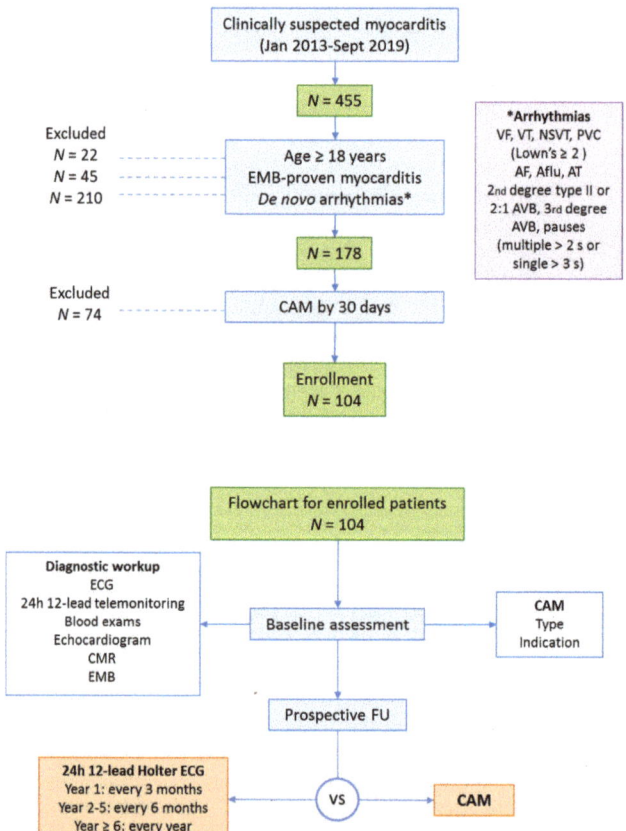

Figure 1. Study flowchart: study design with inclusion criteria is shown. AF = atrial fibrillation; AFlu = atrial flutter; AT = atrial tachycardia; AVB = atrioventricular blocks; CAM = continuous arrhythmia monitoring; CMR = cardiac magnetic resonance; EMB = endomyocardial biopsy; FU = follow up; NSVT = nonsustained ventricular tachycardia; PVC = premature ventricular complexes; VA = ventricular arrhythmia; VF = ventricular fibrillation; VT = ventricular tachycardia.

As part of the baseline diagnostic work-up, all patients underwent complete blood exams, continuous 12-lead ECG telemonitoring, transthoracic echocardiogram and cardiac magnetic resonance (CMR).

2.2. Definitions

Arrhythmias were defined based on updated standards [8–10] and classified into VA, SVA and BA. In detail, VA included ventricular fibrillation (VF), tachycardia (VT), nonsustained VT (NSVT) and grade ≥ 2 premature ventricular complexes (PVCs) according to Lown's classification (i.e., >1 PVC/min or >30 PVC/h) [11]; SVA included AF, atrial flutter and atrial tachycardia; BA included 2nd degree type II, 2:1, or 3rd degree atrioventricular blocks (AVBs) and pauses >3 s. Further definitions, including details concerning VA characterization, are reported in the Supplementary Materials.

Histological signs of fibrosis, cardiac myocyte hypertrophy and nuclear atypia were used to define "chronically active" rather than true "acute" myocarditis [12,13].

2.3. CAM Selection

In the absence of clear guideline recommendations for patients with chronically active myocarditis [5–7], the choice between ICD and ILR was patient-tailored and guided the experience of a referral center for arrhythmia management [14]. In detail, the following putative risk factors were identified a priori as markers of arrhythmic risk: (1) left ventricular ejection fraction (LVEF) < 35% at baseline echocardiogram; (2) non-lymphocytic histotypes, namely cardiac sarcoidosis and giant cell myocarditis; (3) 2nd or 3rd degree AVB; (4) fast (>180 bpm for at least 10 beats) or recurrent (>3 episodes at telemonitoring) NSVT despite antiarrhythmic therapy; (5) induction of VT or VF at baseline programmed ventricular stimulation (PVS) when applicable; (6) extensive areas of either late gadolinium enhancement (LGE) at CMR (>1 LV wall, or >5 of 17 LV segments) or replacement fibrosis at histology (>50% of tissue samples).

For secondary prevention, the ICD implant was indicated following either VT or VF onset. Otherwise, CAM was proposed to all patients: the decision between the primary prevention ICD and ILR implant was personalized, and guided by the above defined risk factors. Details about CAM programming are reported in the Supplementary Materials.

2.4. Follow-Up

All patients underwent prospective follow-up (FU) reassessment [15] through both CAM and 12-lead 24 h Holter ECGs, according to a defined schedule (4/year in the first year; 2/year in years 2–5; and then 1/year). Both in-person and remote monitoring were allowed for CAM, and the arrhythmia timeline was defined by the real event date. The association with symptoms was assessed both by the analysis of manually activated device alerts, and by direct patient interrogation.

2.5. Endpoints

VA occurrence, burden and timing—as detected by CAM vs. Holter ECG monitoring—were analyzed as the primary study endpoint. During FU, appropriate ICD interventions (anti-tachycardia pacing or shock) also constituted VT events. The occurrence of other arrhythmias (SVA, BA) constituted the secondary endpoints. In addition, the appropriateness of the ICD implantation strategy was retrospectively evaluated.

2.6. Statistical Analysis

SPSS Version 20 (IBM Corp., Armonk, NY, USA) was used for the analysis, and Prism Version 6 (GraphPad Software Inc., La Jolla, CA, USA) was used for graphic presentations. Continuous variables were expressed as the mean and standard deviation, or as median and IQR of 25th to 75th percentiles, depending on the distribution of data. Accordingly, continuous variables were compared by Student's t-test or by Mann–Whitney U-test. Categorical variables, reported as counts and percentages, were compared by the Fisher exact test. Cox regression and Kaplan–Meier curves were used for event rate analyses. Where relevant, 2-sided p-values < 0.05 were set as statistically significant. Confidence intervals were set at 95%.

3. Results

3.1. Baseline Characteristics of the Population

Overall, 104 patients (71% males, mean age 47 ± 11 year) were enrolled, including those with arrhythmic presentation (n = 70) and those with arrhythmias detected during in-hospital telemonitoring (n = 34). Patients' complete characteristics are shown in Table 1. Arrhythmias included VAs, SVAs and BAs in 104 (100%), 11 (11%), and 9 patients (9%), respectively. Overall, 19 patients (18%) had LVEF < 35% at presentation. EMB identified 73 cases of chronically active myocarditis (70%) and CMR showed anteroseptal LGE in 26 cases (25%).

Table 1. Baseline characteristics of the population.

Parameter	Units	Total N = 104
Clinical data		
Age (year)	Mean ± SD	47 ± 11
Sex (male)	N (%)	74 (71)
Caucasian	N (%)	98 (94)
Presentation		
ACS-like	N (%)	14 (13)
HF	N (%)	20 (19)
Arrhythmias	N (%)	70 (67)
Family history of SCD/CMP	N (%)	6 (6)
Fever in last 30 days	N (%)	35 (34)
Syncope	N (%)	37 (36)
Palpitation	N (%)	72 (69)
Chest pain	N (%)	25 (24)
Dyspnea	N (%)	40 (38)
NYHA class	Median (IQR)	1 (1–2)
Blood exams		
WBC (10^3/mm^3)	Mean ± SD	8.5 ± 3.5
Neutrophils (%)	Mean ± SD	63 ± 12
CRP (mg/L; n.v. < 6)	Median (IQR)	3.2 (1.5–8.8)
T-Tn (ng/L; n.v. < 14)	Median (IQR)	40 (9–456)
NTproBNP (pg/mL; n.v. < 125)	Median (IQR)	198 (82–843)
ECG		
HR (min^{-1})	Mean ± SD	76 ± 22
PQ (ms)	Mean ± SD	173 ± 28
QRS (ms)	Mean ± SD	103 ± 21
QTc (ms)	Mean ± SD	423 ± 34
Abnormal T waves	N (%)	59 (57)
Abnormal ST	N (%)	30 (29)
Telemonito		
Total VA	N (%)	104 (100)
PVC	N (%)	102 (98)
PVC daily number	Median (IQR)	1201 (209–3390)
NSVT	N (%)	43 (41)
VT	N (%)	39 (38)
VF	N (%)	8 (8)

Table 1. *Cont.*

Parameter	Units	Total N = 104
Total SVA	N (%)	11 (11)
AF	N (%)	9 (9)
Atrial flutter	N (%)	1 (1)
Atrial tachycardia	N (%)	4 (4)
NSAT	N (%)	5 (5)
Total BA	N (%)	9 (9)
Pauses > 3 s	N (%)	3 (3)
1st degree AVB	N (%)	15 (14)
2nd degree AVB Mobitz 1	N (%)	1 (1)
2nd degree AVB Mobitz 2	N (%)	2 (2)
2nd degree AVB 2:1	N (%)	1 (1)
3rd degree AVB	N (%)	6 (6)
Echocard		
LV EDVi (mL/m^2)	Mean ± SD	68 ± 20
LV EF (%)	Mean ± SD	50 ± 13
Regional WMA	N (%)	59 (57)
E/E'	Mean ± SD	8 ± 3
RV EDD (mm)	Mean ± SD	32 ± 4
TAPSE (mm)	Mean ± SD	22 ± 4
SPAP > 30 mmHg	N (%)	8 (8)
Pericardial effusion	N (%)	11 (11)
CMR		
Active myocarditis	N (%)	77 (74)
Classic Lake Louise criteria	N (%)	49 (47)
STIR	N (%)	53 (55)
EGE	N (%)	10 (10)
LGE	N (%)	92 (88)
Abnormal T1-mapping	Fraction	35/41
Abnormal T2-mapping	Fraction	29/41
EMB		
Lymphocytic	N (%)	98 (94)
Eosinophilic	N (%)	0 (0)
Sarcoidosis	N (%)	5 (5)
Giant cell	N (%)	1 (1)
Viral genome	N (%)	18 (17)

Baseline characteristics of the population are shown. ACS = acute coronary syndrome; AF = atrial fibrillation; AVB = atrioventricular block; BA = bradyarrhythmia; CMP = cardiomyopathy; CRP = C-reactive protein; EDD = end-diastolic diameter; EDVi = end-diastolic volume (indexed); EF = ejection fraction; EGE = early gadolinium enhancement; HF = heart failure; HR = heart rate; IQR = interquartile range; LGE = late gadolinium enhancement; LV = left ventricle; n.v. = normal value; NSAT = nonsustained atrial tachyarrhythmia; NSVT = nonsustained ventricular tachycardia; PVC = premature ventricular complexes; RV = right ventricle; SCD = sudden cardiac death; SD = standard deviation; SVA = supraventricular arrhythmias; T-Tn = T troponin; TAPSE = triscupid annular plane systolic excursion; VA = ventricular arrhythmias; VF = ventricular fibrillation; VT = ventricular tachycardia; WMA = wall motion abnormality.

3.2. CAM Types, Indications and Complications

ICDs were implanted in 62 patients (60%; n = 47 for secondary prevention), including dual-chamber (n = 48), single-chamber (n = 5) and subcutaneous devices (S-ICD, n = 9). The remaining 42 patients (40%) underwent ILR implant. The mean number of risk factors was two in ICD carriers and <1 in ILR cases (Table S1). Among the 61 patients undergoing PVS, 25 had VT or VF inducibility and underwent ICD implant (Table S2). Complications were documented in 9/62 ICD carriers (15%) including infection (n = 3), catheter dislocation or malfunctioning ($n = 3$), hematoma ($n = 2$) and pneumothorax ($n = 1$). No complications occurred following ILR implants.

3.3. Treatment and Follow Up

All patients were discharged on medical treatment, including RAAS-inhibitors ($n = 87$), betablockers ($n = 96$), and either single ($n = 47$) or combined ($n = 23$) antiarrhythmic drug (AAD) therapy (Table S3).

The study FU was 3.7 ± 1.6 year. There were no patients lost to FU. The average number of Holter ECGs per patient was 9.5, and the proportion of missed exams was 3.6% (maximum one exam per patient). Three patients died (end-stage heart failure, $n = 1$; infectious complications of cardiac transplantation, $n = 1$; malignancy, $n = 1$), all of which were ICD carriers (guideline-driven implant in two of them). No patients experienced systemic embolism or hemorrhagic complications.

During FU, CMR was repeated in 40 cases (38%), and its interpretation was limited by susceptibility artifacts in all ICD ($n = 5$) and no ILR carriers ($n = 35$, 28 of whom were proven healed from myocarditis). All devices were replaced following the end-of-life status. No quality-of-life issues were reported by 91% of the device carriers (Table S4).

3.4. VA Detection, Burden and Timing

During FU, 45 patients (43%) underwent VT episodes including $n = 3$ incessant VTs, $n = 10$ electrical storms (≥ 3 shocks/24 h) and $n = 32$ paroxysmal VTs only. In 10/45 cases (22%), there was no prior history of VT. In addition, 67 patients (64%) had NSVT and 102 (98%) PVC. Complete data are reported in Table 2. As compared to Holter ECG, CAM identified more patients either with VT (45 vs. 4, $p < 0.001$) or NSVT (64 vs. 45, $p < 0.001$). Kaplan–Meier curves are shown in Figure 2. All VT episodes and most of the NSVT ones were only detected by CAM (Table 2); in addition, CAM allowed earlier NSVT detection (median 6, IQR 3–24 vs. median 24, IQR 9–36 months, respectively, $p < 0.001$). Event rates are shown in Figure S1.

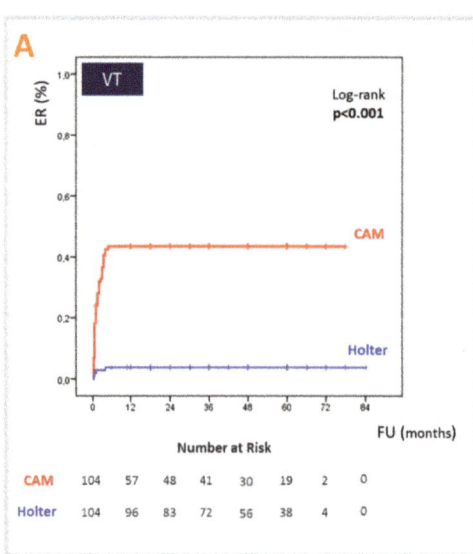
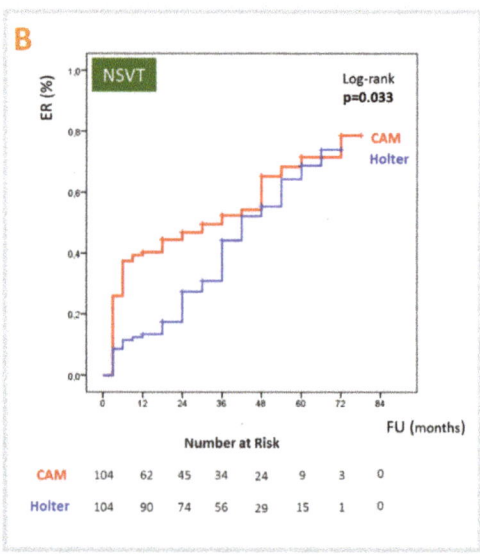

Figure 2. Detection of ventricular arrhythmias by CAM vs. sequential 24 h Holter ECGs. Kaplan–Meier curves are shown for the endpoint of VT (panel **A**) and NSVT (panel **B**). CAM = continuous arrhythmia monitoring (red); ER = event rate; FU = follow up; Holter = 24 h Holter ECG (blue); NSVT = nonsustained ventricular tachycardia; VT = ventricular tachycardia.

Table 2. Arrhythmia detection during follow up.

Arrhythmia Type		Total	De Novo	By Month 12	Technique By Holter	Technique By CAM	p
VT [1]	Patients, N (%)	45	10 (22)	25 (56)	4 (9)	45 (100)	<0.001
	Episodes, N (%)	115	-	44 (38)	5 (4)	115 (100)	-
NSVT	Patients, N (%)	67	27 (40)	44 (66)	45 (67)	64 (95)	<0.001
	Episodes, N (%)	3224	-	1515 (47)	386 (12)	2933 (91)	-
PVC	Patients, N (%)	102	2 (2)	99 (97)	102 (100)	21 (21)	<0.001
	>10^3 daily	71	4 (6)	66 (93)	71 (70)	-	-
AF [2]	Patients, N (%)	19	13 (68)	7 (37)	3 (16)	19 (100)	<0.001
	>24 h	6	6 (100)	2 (33)	0 (0)	6 (100)	0.002
	Episodes, N (%)	45	-	9 (20)	4 (9)	45 (100)	-
	> 24 h	12	-	2 (17)	0 (0)	12 (100)	-
Atrial flutter/AT [2]	Patients, N (%)	11	10 (91)	4 (36)	5 (45)	11 (100)	0.012
	>24 h	3	2 (67)	1 (33)	1 (33)	3 (100)	0.400
	Episodes, N (%)	58	-	13 (22)	10 (17)	58 (100)	-
	> 24 h	4	-	1 (25)	1 (25)	4 (100)	-
NSAT [3]	Patients, N (%)	43	38 (88)	20 (47)	17 (40)	43 (100)	<0.001
	Episodes, N (%)	162	-	33 (20)	38 (23)	162 (100)	-
BA [4]	Patients, N (%)	6	4 (67)	3 (50)	1 (14)	6 (100)	0.015
	Episodes, N (%)	10	-	4 (40)	1 (10)	9 (90)	-
Pause 2–3 s	Patients, N (%)	18	14 (78)	11 (61)	18 (100)	0 (0)	<0.001
	Episodes, N (%)	24	-	12 (50)	24 (100)	0 (0)	-

Arrhythmia types documented during follow up are shown as detected by Holter ECG vs. CAM. Both the number of episodes and the number of patients are reported: [1] VT includes sustained VT and appropriate ICD therapy (either ATP or shock); [2] AF and AT only include episodes lasting > 30 s; [3] NSAT includes supraventricular arrhythmia episodes lasting $\leq$ 30 s; [4] BA includes 2nd type II, 2:1 or 3rd degree atrioventricular blocks and pauses > 3 s. AF = atrial fibrillation (paroxysmal); AT = atrial tachycardia; ATP = anti-tachycardia pacing; BA = bradyarrhythmia; CAM = continuous arrhythmia monitoring; ICD = implantable cardioverter defibrillator; NSAT = nonsustained atrial tachyarrhythmia; NSVT = nonsustained ventricular tachycardia; PVC = premature ventricular complex; VT = ventricular tachycardia.

Although an alert for clustered PVC was reported by CAM in 21 cases (21%), PVCs were documented by Holter ECG in 102/102 patients ($p < 0.001$). During FU, CAM showed a significant reduction in VT/NSVT cycle length variability, whereas the Holter ECG documented a progressive prevalence of monomorphic PVC (Figure S2).

3.5. Other Arrhythmias

During FU, SVA episodes were documented in 27 patients (26%) including AF in 19 cases (18%). In addition, six patients had BA, mainly second- and third-degree AVB. Complete data are shown in Table 2. Overall, CAM identified more patients either with SVA lasting > 24 h (9 vs. 1, $p < 0.001$), or BA (6 vs. 1, $p = 0.015$) and only missed pauses in the range of 2–3 s. SVA detection by CAM was earlier than that by Holter ECG (22 $\pm$ 8 months in 27 patients vs. 36 $\pm$ 12 months in 7 patients, respectively, $p = 0.001$).

3.6. CAM Type and Indication

Arrhythmia recordings in different CAM subgroups are shown in Table S5. Although most VA occurred in patients following secondary prevention ICD implant, VTs were also documented within primary prevention ICD (10 episodes in $n = 8$ patients) and ILR subgroups (two episodes in two patients).

A FU VT was found in 40/80 patients with putative risk factors vs. 5/24 without putative risk factors (HR 3.8, 95% CI 1.3–11.2, $p = 0.015$). However, there was no a single risk factor capable of predicting the occurrence of a de novo VT (Table 3). Instead, our post hoc analysis identified both anteroseptal LGE distribution pattern at CMR, and signs of chronically active myocarditis at EMB, as significantly associated with the first episode of VT during FU (respectively: 50 vs. 13% and 90 vs. 49%, both $p < 0.05$). Results were confirmed for the whole study cohort, where VT episodes were more common in the chronically active myocarditis and anteroseptal LGE subgroups (respectively: 40/73 vs. 5/31 acute cases, $p < 0.001$; and 16/26 vs. 29/78 inferolateral cases, $p = 0.04$).

Table 3. Characteristics of primary prevention CAM patients with follow-up VT vs. without follow-up VT.

	Units	VT+ N = 10	VT− N = 47	p
Putative risk factors				
LVEF < 35%	N (%)	3 (30)	15 (32)	1.000
Granulomatous	N (%)	1 (10)	1 (2)	0.323
2nd/3rd degree AVB	N (%)	1 (10)	5 (11)	1.000
Fast/recurrent NSVT	N (%)	1 (10)	4 (9)	1.000
Positive PVS	N (%)	1 (10)	0 (0)	0.174
Extensive LGE or fibrosis *	N (%)	3 (30)	18 (38)	0.730
Other baseline features				
Sex (male)	N (%)	8 (80)	32 (68)	0.706
Age > 40 year	N (%)	6 (60)	26 (55)	1.000
SVA	N (%)	2 (20)	3 (6)	0.208
LVEF < 50%	N (%)	7 (70)	19 (40)	0.160
Anteroseptal LGE	N (%)	5 (50)	6 (13)	**0.016**
Chronically active myocarditis	N (%)	9 (90)	23 (49)	**0.031**

Characteristics of the 10 patients experiencing their first VT episode (VT+) during follow up are shown. Significant differences are evidenced in bold. * The definition includes extensive areas of LGE (>1 left ventricular wall, or >5 of 17 left ventricular segments) at cardiac magnetic resonance, or replacement fibrosis in >50% of endomyocardial samples undergoing histological analysis. AVB = atrioventricular blocks; CAM = continuous arrhythmia monitoring; ILR = implantable loop recorder; LGE = late gadolinium enhancement; LVEF = left ventricular ejection fraction; NSVT = nonsustained ventricular tachycardia; PVS = programmed ventricular stimulation; VT = ventricular tachycardia.

3.7. Clinical Impact

Guided by CAM for VT episodes and by Holter ECG for high-burden PVCs, 41 patients (39%) underwent transcatheter ablation during FU. Apart from the VT episodes, most FU arrhythmias were asymptomatic (Table S6). Significantly, de novo oral anticoagulants were started in eight SVA patients (8%) including six asymptomatic ILR carriers. An upgrade to dual-chamber ICD was performed in eight cases (8%) including ILR patients ($n = 5$; two for VT and three for NSVT associated with BA), and ICD cases experiencing inappropriate shocks for AF ($n = 3$; two single-chamber ICDs and one S-ICD).

Based on the current guideline recommendations [5,6], only the five patients with granulomatous myocarditis (5%) and VT/VF onset would have met the criteria for an early ICD implant. However, among the 99 candidates for an ICD-sparing strategy, 41 (41%) experienced at least one VT episode during FU. By the end of the study, the ICD implantation strategy was appropriate in 80% of the population instead of 60%, resulting from the strict application of the guidelines (Figure 3).

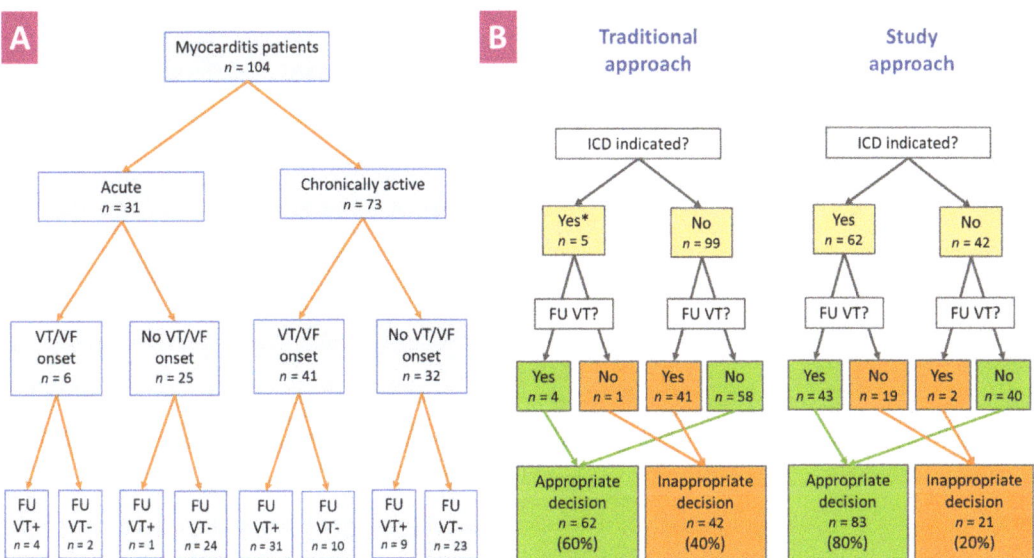

Figure 3. Events by myocarditis stage and implantation strategy. Panel **A**: VT events (VT+) in patients with true acute vs. chronically active myocarditis according to endomyocardial biopsy findings; Panel **B**: Appropriateness of the ICD implantation strategy by application of current guidelines for acute myocarditis (left panel) vs. by multiparametric approach as described in this study (right panel). FU = follow up; ICD = implantable cardioverter defibrillator; VF = ventricular fibrillation; VT = ventricular tachycardia.

4. Discussion

4.1. Major Findings

We described the first study aimed at exploring the advantages of CAM as compared to standard Holter ECG monitoring in patients with EMB-proven active myocarditis [5,13] and evidence of arrhythmias at index hospitalization. Remarkably, the comparison between techniques was unbiased since all patients underwent both CAM and Holter monitoring strategies. Despite the considerable number of Holter ECG exams per patient, we showed that CAM was more accurate in both detecting and quantifying most of the clinically impactful arrhythmias. In addition, we showed that despite a uniform clinical presentation with acute myocarditis [5,6], many patients had histopathological signs suggesting chronically active disease [4,14]: in light of the significant association with follow-up VT episodes, an earlier indication of the ICD implant could be considered for the latter ones.

4.2. Diagnostic Accuracy for VA

As shown in Table 2, all FU VT episodes were detected by CAM. Compared to Holter ECG, CAM was superior in both identifying patients with VA and detecting total VA episodes. Although more frequently detected by ICDs, VA episodes were also found in a relevant proportion of ILR carriers (Table S5). Conversely, the CAM accuracy in detecting PVCs was remarkably lower compared to Holter ECG, which allowed precise PVC quantification over time [10]. As a relevant guidance for the planning of catheter ablation strategies, the clinical VA morphology requires documentation by 12-lead ECG recording [10,16]. Recently, VA characterization by ECG has also been proposed as a tool to assess the myocardial inflammatory stage [17,18] and identify the suitable candidates for VT ablation [16]. In keeping with myocarditis healing, CAM recordings documented a progressive reduction in VA cycle length variability during follow-up, in parallel with a prevalence of monomorphic PVC by Holter ECG (Figure S2).

4.3. Other Arrhythmias

Table 2 shows that CAM was an accurate tool also for diagnosing SVA and BA. Remarkably, most of the long-lasting SVAs were those which were late onset (Figure S1) and asymptomatic (Table S6). In this setting, the CAM-guided anticoagulation strategy [19] was safe since no ischemic or hemorrhagic complications occurred. In turn, advanced AVBs, commonly reported in acute-phase cardiac sarcoidosis [4], were documented even later during FU. Although iatrogenic effects from betablockers and AADs were likely (Table S3), the documentation of both BA and NSVT constituted an indication to ICD upgrading in three ILR carriers (Table S6). Instead, the possible underdiagnosis of BA in transvenous ICD carriers constituted a clinically neglectable issue.

4.4. Arrhythmic Risk Estimation

In our study, the indication of ICD was supported by a number of pre-selected risk factors, namely: LVEF < 35% [6,7]; malignant histotypes [4]; major BA [9]; fast/recurrent NSVT [10]; positive PVS [20]; and extensive LGE or myocardial fibrosis [21,22]. Although VT events more commonly occurred in patients with at least one of the above risk factors, none of the candidates were able to predict an adverse outcome in primary prevention. In keeping with prior studies, we identified anteroseptal LGE [23–26] and histological signs suggesting chronic myocarditis [12,13] as factors associated with adverse arrhythmic outcomes, both in the whole cohort and in patients without malignant VA onset. Results are consistent with recently published data [27]. As suggested by Table 3, mild systolic dysfunction (i.e., LVEF < 50%) may play an additional role for primary prevention risk stratification, as already suggested both in myocarditis and other cardiomyopathies [28,29].

4.5. Device Indication and Choice

Overall, our data challenge the uniform application of an ICD-sparing strategy in patients with VA onset and newly diagnosed active myocarditis [5,6]. Actually, our analysis revealed that, despite the clinically acute myocarditis onset, the majority of patients in our cohort had histological signs of chronic myocarditis, as supported by myocardial fibrosis and additional cellular abnormalities [12,13]. In contrast to the truly "acute" myocarditis cases, those with "chronically active" inflammation showed a significantly higher occurrence of VT during FU—even in the absence of granulomatous myocarditis (Figure 3). Our findings indicate that clinical guidelines may benefit from a clear distinction between the scenarios, and we suggest that a multiparametric assessment could be implemented in chronic setting to identify the most suitable candidates for an early ICD implant [14].

As for the device choice, in our experience, dual-chamber ICDs are advisable to minimize the risk of inappropriate shocks by single-lead devices. In turn, since scar-related VA may even occur during the post-inflammatory stage of myocarditis [16,17], the use of wearable cardioverter defibrillators could be undermined by the unpredictable optimal timing for device withdrawal: while life-vests are currently recommended as a bridge for decision making in acute myocarditis [5,30], S-ICDs may constitute a valuable alternative in the chronic setting. Finally, because of a combination of high diagnostic accuracy, general acceptance among patients (Table S4) and CMR feasibility [31,32], we suggest the widespread use of ILRs as optimal diagnostic tools for the remaining low-risk patients with arrhythmic myocarditis [33,34].

4.6. Study Limitations

Our study specifically focused on patients with myocarditis and the evidence of VA at the index of hospitalization. Although the arrhythmic population is underinvestigated and clinically demanding [4–7], results should not be inappropriately generalized to different clinical scenarios. Selection bias related to the center experience [14,33] as well as baseline arrhythmia overdetection due the use of continuous in-hospital telemonitoring should be taken into account. Importantly, CAM choice was conditioned by a number of risk factors that, although reasonable, were not supported by robust evidence—this introduces a bias by indication. Baseline PVS was not performed in all patients, and wearable devices were not hereby investigated. Finally, some differences in arrhythmia detection capability should be considered for ICDs (unable to detect BA unless permanent pacing is needed) and for single-chamber and subcutaneous devices (which may be less reliable in differentiating SVA and VA subtypes). Larger prospective multicenter studies are needed to validate our findings and improve patient selection for each device type at different inflammatory stages [16–18].

5. Conclusions

In patients with arrhythmic myocarditis, CAM was a clinically useful tool to detect arrhythmias and guide relevant therapeutical decisions. As compared to sequential Holter ECGs, CAM allowed an earlier detection and greater diagnostic yield for most arrhythmias. As a complementary tool, Holter ECG allowed PVC quantification and morphology characterization. Based on our findings, efforts are needed to identify patients with chronically active myocarditis, as well as those with anteroseptal LGE at CMR, who may benefit from an earlier ICD implant. In low-risk patients, ILR was a feasible and sensitive diagnostic tool, allowing also to monitor myocarditis evolution by informative CMR. Prospective controlled trials including appropriate myocarditis staging and a uniform implantation strategy are needed, to improve the arrhythmic risk stratification and patient selection for different device types.

Supplementary Materials: The following are available online at https://www.mdpi.com/article/10.3390/jcm10215142/s1, Supplementary Materials. Table S1: Indications to different CAM types; Table S2: Programmed ventricular stimulation; Table S3: Treatment; Table S4: Quality of life; Table S5: Arrhythmia detection according to CAM type and indication; Table S6: Clinical impact of arrhythmia detection; Figure S1: Arrhythmic event rates; Figure S2: VA modifications during follow-up.

Author Contributions: Conceptualization, G.P. (Giovanni Peretto) and S.S.; methodology, G.P. (Gabriele Paglino), P.M., A.M., G.T., S.R. and C.B.; validation, P.M. and P.D.B.; formal analysis, G.P. (Giovanni Peretto); investigation, G.P. (Giovanni Peretto) and S.S.; resources, P.D.B.; data curation, G.P. (Giovanni Peretto), G.T. and A.M.; writing—original draft preparation, G.P. (Giovanni Peretto); writing—review and editing, S.S.; visualization, G.P. (Giovanni Peretto), P.M., G.P. (Gabriele Paglino), A.M., G.T., S.R., C.B., P.D.B. and S.S. All authors have read and agreed to the published version of the manuscript.

Funding: This research received no external funding.

Institutional Review Board Statement: This study was conducted according to the guidelines of the Declaration of Helsinki and approved by the Institutional Review Board of San Raffaele Scientific Institute (MYOCAR, 24/01/2018).

Informed Consent Statement: Informed consent was obtained from all subjects involved in the study.

Data Availability Statement: Data will be made available, upon reasonable request, by emailing the correspondent author.

Conflicts of Interest: The authors declare no conflict of interest regarding the publication of this manuscript.

Abbreviations

AAD	antiarrhythmic drug
AF	atrial fibrillation
AVB	atrioventricular block
BA	bradyarrhythmia
CAM	continuous arrhythmia monitoring

CMR	cardiac magnetic resonance
EMB	endomyocardial biopsy
FU	follow up
ICD	implantable cardioverter defibrillator
ILR	implantable loop recorder
LGE	late gadolinium enhancement
LVEF	left ventricular ejection fraction
NSAT	nonsustained atrial tachyarrhythmia
NSVT	nonsustained ventricular tachycardia
PVC	premature ventricular complexes
PVS	programmed ventricular stimulation
SVA	supraventricular arrhythmias
VA	ventricular arrhythmias
VT	ventricular tachycardia

References

1. Giancaterino, S.; Lupercio, F.; Nishimura, M.; Hsu, J.C. Current and Future Use of Insertable Cardiac Monitors. *JACC Clin. Electrophysiol.* **2018**, *4*, 1383–1396. [CrossRef]
2. Long-Term Continuous Ambulatory ECG Monitors and External Cardiac Loop Recorders for Cardiac Arrhythmia: A Health Technology Assessment Health Quality Ontario. *Ont. Health Technol. Assess. Ser.* **2017**, *17*, 1–56.
3. Steinberg, J.S.; Varma, N.; Cygankiewicz, I.; Aziz, P.; Balsam, P.; Baranchuk, A.; Cantillon, D.J.; Dilaveris, P.; Dubner, S.J.; El-Sherif, N.; et al. 2017 ISHNE-HRS expert consensus statement on ambulatory ECG and external cardiac monitoring/telemetry. *Heart Rhythm.* **2017**, *14*, e55–e96. [CrossRef]
4. Peretto, G.; Sala, S.; Rizzo, S.; De Luca, G.; Campochiaro, C.; Sartorelli, S.; Benedetti, G.; Palmisano, A.; Esposito, A.; Tresoldi, M.; et al. Arrhythmias in myocarditis: State of the art. *Heart Rhythm.* **2019**, *16*, 793–801. [CrossRef]
5. Caforio, A.L.P.; Pankuweit, S.; Arbustini, E.; Basso, C.; Blanes, J.G.; Felix, S.B.; Fu, M.; Heliö, T.; Heymans, S.; Jahns, R.; et al. Current state of knowledge on aetiology, diagnosis, management, and therapy of myocarditis: A position statement of the European Society of Cardiology Working Group on Myocardial and Pericardial Diseases. *Eur. Heart J.* **2013**, *34*, 2636–2648. [CrossRef]
6. Task Force Members; Priori, S.G.; Blomström-Lundqvist, C.; Mazzanti, A.; Blom, N.; Borggrefe, M.; Zannad, F. 2015 ESC Guidelines for the management of patients with ventricular arrhythmias and the prevention of sudden cardiac death. *Europace* **2015**, *17*, 1601–1687.
7. Al-Khatib, S.M.; Stevenson, W.G.; Ackerman, M.J.; Bryant, W.J.; Callans, D.J.; Curtis, A.B.; Deal, B.J.; Dickfeld, T.; Field, M.E.; Fonarow, G.C.; et al. 2017 AHA/ACC/HRS guideline for management of patients with ventricular arrhythmias and the prevention of sudden cardiac death. *Heart Rhythm.* **2018**, *15*, e190–e252. [CrossRef]
8. January, C.T.; Wann, L.S.; Calkins, H.; Chen, L.Y.; Cigarroa, J.E.; Cleveland, J.C., Jr.; Ellinor, P.T.; Ezekowitz, M.D.; Field, M.E.; Furie, K.L.; et al. 2019 AHA/ACC/HRS Focused Update of the 2014 AHA/ACC/HRS Guideline for the Management of Patients with Atrial Fibrillation: A Report of the American College of Cardiology/American Heart Association Task Force on Clinical Practice Guidelines and the Heart Rhythm Society in Collaboration With the Society of Thoracic Surgeons. *Circulation* **2019**, *140*, e125–e151. [CrossRef]
9. Kusumoto, F.M.; Schoenfeld, M.H.; Barrett, C.; Edgerton, J.R.; Ellenbogen, K.A.; Gold, M.R.; Goldschlager, N.F.; Hamilton, R.M.; Joglar, J.A.; Kim, R.J.; et al. 2018 ACC/AHA/HRS Guideline on the Evaluation and Management of Patients with Bradycardia and Cardiac Conduction Delay: A Report of the American College of Cardiology/American Heart Association Task Force on Clinical Practice Guidelines and the Heart Rhythm Society. *J. Am. Coll. Cardiol.* **2019**, *74*, e151–e156.
10. Cronin, E.M.; Bogun, F.M.; Maury, P.; Peichl, P.; Chen, M.; Namboodiri, N.; Aguinaga, L.; Leite, L.R.; Al-Khatib, S.M.; Anter, E.; et al. 2019 HRS/EHRA/APHRS/LAHRS expert consensus statement on catheter ablation of ventricular arrhythmias: Executive summary. *Europace* **2020**, *22*, 450–495. [CrossRef]
11. Lown, B.; Wolf, M. Approaches to Sudden Death from Coronary Heart Disease. *Circulation* **1971**, *44*, 130–142. [CrossRef]
12. Leone, O.; Veinot, J.P.; Angelini, A.; Baandrup, U.T.; Basso, C.; Berry, G.; Bruneval, P.; Burke, M.; Butany, J.; Calabrese, F.; et al. 2011 Consensus statement on endomyocardial biopsy from the Association for European Cardiovascular Pathology and the Society for Cardiovascular Pathology. *Cardiovasc. Pathol.* **2012**, *21*, 245–274. [CrossRef]
13. Ammirati, E.; Frigerio, M.; Adler, E.D.; Basso, C.; Birnie, D.H.; Brambatti, M.; Friedrich, M.G.; Klingel, K.; Lehtonen, J.; Moslehi, J.J.; et al. Management of Acute Myocarditis and Chronic Inflammatory Cardiomyopathy: An Expert Consensus Document. *Circ. Heart Fail.* **2020**, *13*, e007405. [CrossRef]
14. Peretto, G.; Sala, S.; Della Bella, P. Diagnostic and therapeutic approach to myocarditis patients presenting with arrhythmias. *G. Ital. Cardiol.* **2020**, *21*, 187–194.

15. Peretto, G.; De Luca, G.; Campochiaro, C.; Palmisano, A.; Busnardo, E.; Sartorelli, S.; Barzaghi, F.; Cicalese, M.P.; Esposito, A.; Sala, S. Telemedicine in myocarditis: Evolution of a mutidisciplinary "disease unit" at the time of COVID-19 pandemic. *Am. Heart J.* **2020**, *229*, 121–126. [CrossRef]
16. Peretto, G.; Sala, S.; Basso, C.; Rizzo, S.; Radinovic, A.; Frontera, A.; Limite, L.R.; Paglino, G.; Bisceglia, C.; De Luca, G.; et al. Inflammation as a Predictor of Recurrent Ventricular Tachycardia after Ablation in Patients with Myocarditis. *J. Am. Coll. Cardiol.* **2020**, *76*, 1644–1656. [CrossRef]
17. Peretto, G.; Sala, S.; Rizzo, S.; Palmisano, A.; Esposito, A.; De Cobelli, F.; Campochiaro, C.; De Luca, G.; Foppoli, L.; Dagna, L.; et al. Ventricular Arrhythmias in Myocarditis: Characterization and Relationships with Myocardial Inflammation. *J. Am. Coll. Cardiol.* **2020**, *75*, 1046–1057. [CrossRef]
18. Peretto, G.; Sala, S.; De Luca, G.; Marcolongo, R.; Campochiaro, C.; Sartorelli, S.; Tresoldi, M.; Foppoli, L.; Palmisano, A.; Esposito, A.; et al. Immunosuppressive Therapy and Risk Stratification of Patients with Myocarditis Presenting with Ventricular Arrhythmias. *JACC Clin. Electrophysiol.* **2020**, *6*, 1221–1234. [CrossRef]
19. Matos, J.; Waks, J.; Zimetbaum, P. Tailored Anticoagulation for Thromboembolic Risk Reduction in Paroxysmal Atrial Fibrillation. *J. Innov. Card. Rhythm. Manag.* **2018**, *9*, 3116–3125. [CrossRef]
20. Peretto, G.; Sala, S.; Basso, C.; Della Bella, P. Programmed ventricular stimulation in patients with active vs previous arrhythmic myocarditis. *J. Cardiovasc. Electrophysiol.* **2020**, *31*, 692–701. [CrossRef]
21. Zorzi, A.; Marra, M.P.; Rigato, I.; De Lazzari, M.; Susana, A.; Niero, A.; Pilichou, K.; Migliore, F.; Rizzo, S.; Giorgi, B.; et al. Nonischemic Left Ventricular Scar as a Substrate of Life-Threatening Ventricular Arrhythmias and Sudden Cardiac Death in Competitive Athletes. *Circ. Arrhythmia Electrophysiol.* **2016**, *9*, e004229. [CrossRef]
22. Peretto, G.; Sala, S.; De Luca, G.; Campochiaro, C.; Sartorelli, S.; Cappelletti, A.M.; Rizzo, S.; Palmisano, A.; Esposito, A.; Margonato, A.; et al. Impact of systemic immune-mediated diseases on clinical features and prognosis of patients with biopsy-proved myocarditis. *Int. J. Cardiol.* **2019**, *280*, 110–116. [CrossRef]
23. Aquaro, G.D.; Perfetti, M.; Camastra, G.; Monti, L.; Dellegrottaglie, S.; Moro, C.; Pepe, A.; Todiere, G.; Lanzillo, C.; Scatteia, A.; et al. Cardiac MR with Late Gadolinium Enhancement in Acute Myocarditis with Preserved Systolic Function: ITAMY Study. *J. Am. Coll. Cardiol.* **2017**, *70*, 1977–1987. [CrossRef]
24. Oloriz, T.; Wellens, H.J.; Santagostino, G.; Trevisi, N.; Silberbauer, J.; Peretto, G.; Maccabelli, G.; Della Bella, P. The value of the 12-lead electrocardiogram in localizing the scar in non-ischaemic cardiomyopathy. *Europace* **2016**, *18*, 1850–1859. [CrossRef]
25. Peretto, G.; Sala, S.; Lazzeroni, D.; Palmisano, A.; Gigli, L.; Esposito, A.; De Cobelli, F.; Camici, P.G.; Mazzone, P.; Basso, C.; et al. Septal Late Gadolinium Enhancement and Arrhythmic Risk in Genetic and Acquired Non-Ischaemic Cardiomyopathies. *Hear. Lung Circ.* **2020**, *29*, 1356–1365. [CrossRef]
26. Casella, M.; Bergonti, M.; Narducci, M.L.; Persampieri, S.; Gasperetti, A.; Conte, E.; Catto, V.; Carbucicchio, C.; Guerra, F.; Pontone, G.; et al. Prior myocarditis and ventricular arrhythmias: The importance of scar pattern. *Heart Rhythm.* **2020**, *18*, 589–596. [CrossRef]
27. Gentile, P.; Merlo, M.; Peretto, G.; Ammirati, E.; Sala, S.; Della Bella, P.; Aquaro, G.D.; Imazio, M.; Potena, L.; Campodonico, J.; et al. Post-discharge arrhythmic risk stratification of patients with acute myocarditis and life-threatening ventricular tachyarrhythmias. *Eur. J. Heart Fail.* **2021**. [CrossRef]
28. Ammirati, E.; Cipriani, M.; Moro, C.; Raineri, C.; Pini, D.; Sormani, P.; Mantovani, R.; Varrenti, M.; Pedrotti, P.; Conca, C.; et al. Clinical Presentation and Outcome in a Contemporary Cohort of Patients with Acute Myocarditis: Multicenter Lombardy Registry. *Circulation* **2018**, *138*, 1088–1099. [CrossRef]
29. Peretto, G.; Di Resta, C.; Perversi, J.; Forleo, C.; Maggi, L.; Politano, L.; Barison, A.; Previtali, S.C.; Carboni, N.; Brun, F.; et al. Cardiac and Neuromuscular Features of Patients WithLMNA-Related Cardiomyopathy. *Ann. Intern. Med.* **2019**, *171*, 458. [CrossRef]
30. Peretto, G.; Barzaghi, F.; Cicalese, M.P.; Di Resta, C.; Slavich, M.; Benedetti, S.; Giangiobbe, S.; Rizzo, S.; Palmisano, A.; Esposito, A.; et al. Immunosuppressive therapy in childhood-onset arrhythmogenic inflammatory cardiomyopathy. *Pacing Clin. Electrophysiol.* **2021**, *44*, 552–556. [CrossRef] [PubMed]
31. Aquaro, G.D.; Habtemicael, Y.G.; Camastra, G.; Monti, L.; Dellegrottaglie, S.; Moro, C.; Lanzillo, C.; Scatteia, A.; Di Roma, M.; Pontone, G.; et al. Prognostic Value of Repeating Cardiac Magnetic Resonance in Patients with Acute Myocarditis. *J. Am. Coll. Cardiol.* **2019**, *74*, 2439–2448. [CrossRef] [PubMed]
32. Palmisano, A.; Vignale, D.; Peretto, G.; Busnardo, E.; Calcagno, C.; Campochiaro, C.; De Luca, G.; Sala, S.; Ferro, P.; Basso, C.; et al. Hybrid FDG-PET/MR or FDG-PET/CT to Detect Disease Activity in Patients with Persisting Arrhythmias after Myocarditis. *JACC Cardiovasc. Imaging* **2021**, *14*, 288–292. [CrossRef] [PubMed]
33. Mazzone, P.; Peretto, G.; Radinovic, A.; Limite, L.R.; Marzi, A.; Sala, S.; Cireddu, M.; Vegara, P.; Baratto, F.; Paglino, G.; et al. The COVID-19 challenge to cardiac electrophysiologists: Optimizing resources at a referral center. *J. Interv. Card. Electrophysiol.* **2020**, *59*, 321–327. [CrossRef] [PubMed]
34. Peretto, G.; Villatore, A.; Rizzo, S.; Esposito, A.; De Luca, G.; Palmisano, A.; Vignale, D.; Cappelletti, A.; Tresoldi, M.; Campochiaro, C.; et al. The Spectrum of COVID-19-Associated Myocarditis: A Patient-Tailored Multidisciplinary Approach. *J. Clin. Med.* **2021**, *10*, 1974. [CrossRef] [PubMed]

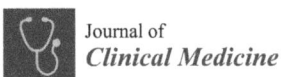

Article

Relationship between Adipokines and Cardiovascular Ultrasound Parameters in Metabolic-Dysfunction-Associated Fatty Liver Disease

Abdulrahman Ismaiel [1], Mihail Spinu [2], Livia Budisan [3], Daniel-Corneliu Leucuta [4], Stefan-Lucian Popa [1,*], Bogdan Augustin Chis [1], Ioana Berindan-Neagoe [3,5,6], Dan Mircea Olinic [2,7] and Dan L. Dumitrascu [1]

[1] 2nd Department of Internal Medicine, "Iuliu Hatieganu" University of Medicine and Pharmacy, 400006 Cluj-Napoca, Romania; abdulrahman.ismaiel@yahoo.com (A.I.); bogdan_a_chis@yahoo.com (B.A.C.); ddumitrascu@umfcluj.ro (D.L.D.)
[2] Medical Clinic No. 1, "Iuliu Hatieganu" University of Medicine and Pharmacy, 400006 Cluj-Napoca, Romania; spinu_mihai@yahoo.com (M.S.); danolinic@gmail.com (D.M.O.)
[3] Research Center for Functional Genomics, Biomedicine and Translational Medicine, "Iuliu Hațieganu" University of Medicine and Pharmacy, 400337 Cluj-Napoca, Romania; lbudisan@yahoo.com (L.B.); ioana.neagoe@umfcluj.ro (I.B.-N.)
[4] Department of Medical Informatics and Biostatistics, "Iuliu Hatieganu" University of Medicine and Pharmacy, 400349 Cluj-Napoca, Romania; dleucuta@umfcluj.ro
[5] Research Center for Advanced Medicine-Medfuture, Iuliu Hatieganu University of Medicine and Pharmacy, 23 Marinescu Street, 400337 Cluj-Napoca, Romania
[6] Department of Functional Genomics and Experimental Pathology, The Oncology Institute "Prof. Dr. Ion Chiricuta", 400015 Cluj-Napoca, Romania
[7] Interventional Cardiology Department, Emergency Clinical Hospital, 400006 Cluj-Napoca, Romania
* Correspondence: popa.stefan@umfcluj.ro; Tel.: +40-755855262

Abstract: (1) Background: The role of adipokines such as adiponectin and visfatin in metabolic-dysfunction-associated fatty liver disease (MAFLD) and cardiovascular disease remains unclear. Therefore, we aim to assess serum adiponectin and visfatin levels in MAFLD patients and associated cardiovascular parameters. (2) Methods: A cross-sectional study involving 80 participants (40 MAFLD patients, 40 controls), recruited between January and September 2020, was conducted, using both hepatic ultrasonography and SteatoTestTM to evaluate hepatic steatosis. Echocardiographic and Doppler parameters were assessed. Serum adipokines were measured using ELISA kits. (3) Results: Adiponectin and visfatin levels were not significantly different in MAFLD vs. controls. Visfatin was associated with mean carotid intima-media thickness (p-value = 0.047), while adiponectin was associated with left ventricular ejection fraction (LVEF) (p-value = 0.039) and E/A ratio (p-value = 0.002) in controls. The association between adiponectin and E/A ratio was significant in the univariate analysis at 95% CI (0.0049–0.1331, p-value = 0.035), but lost significance after the multivariate analysis. Although LVEF was not associated with adiponectin in the univariate analysis, significant values were observed after the multivariate analysis (95% CI (−1.83)–(−0.22), p-value = 0.015). (4) Conclusions: No significant difference in serum adiponectin and visfatin levels in MAFLD patients vs. controls was found. Interestingly, although adiponectin levels were not associated with LVEF in the univariate analysis, a significant inversely proportional association was observed after the multivariate analysis.

Keywords: metabolic-dysfunction-associated fatty liver disease (MAFLD); hepatic steatosis; SteatoTest; adipokines; adiponectin; visfatin; cardiovascular disease

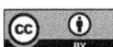

1. Introduction

Although fatty liver disease is mainly associated with structural and functional liver alterations, as well as increased liver-related morbidity and mortality as a result of possible progression to cirrhosis, liver failure and, ultimately, hepatocellular carcinoma, it is also well known to exert several extrahepatic manifestations [1–4]. Lately, a significant increase in the worldwide prevalence of metabolic-dysfunction-associated diseases, including fatty liver disease, type 2 diabetes mellitus, dyslipidemia and obesity, has been documented [5]. Despite the importance of treating fatty liver disease, we still remain without approved pharmacotherapies [6].

Recently, the term metabolic-dysfunction-associated fatty liver disease (MAFLD) was suggested to replace the previously known non-alcoholic fatty liver disease (NAFLD) which is defined by the presence of steatosis in >5% of hepatocytes, associated with insulin resistance (IR) [1,2,7]. On the other hand, MAFLD is defined by the presence of fatty liver, in addition to one of the following three criteria: overweight/obesity, type 2 diabetes mellitus, or confirmed metabolic risk dysregulation [8,9]. Therefore, the terms NAFLD and MAFLD should not be used interchangeably due to the diagnostic criteria differences between the terms. Multiple studies reported fatty liver disease as an independent risk factor associated with increased cardiovascular disease (CVD)-related morbidity and all-cause mortality [10,11]. This association can be attributed to several possible pathogenic factors increasing the CV risk in MAFLD, including IR, systemic inflammation, cytokines, oxidative stress, adipokines, hepatokines, genes and intestinal microbiota [12]. Nevertheless, other studies demonstrated that fatty liver disease per se is not causally related to an increased cardiovascular (CV) risk, implying an essential role of plasma lipids in this relationship.

Interestingly, a recently published study demonstrated that MAFLD was found to be associated with a higher risk for cardiovascular mortality and risk of all-cause mortality [13,14]. However, NAFLD per se did not increase the risk of all-cause deaths after adjusting for metabolic risk factors. Therefore, possible pathogenic factors linking cardiovascular disease to fatty liver disease should be reassessed using the newly defined MAFLD criteria due to possible result differences.

Adipose tissue, known to act as a highly active endocrine tissue, produces peptides known as adipokines with autocrine, paracrine and endocrine functions. Lately, an increased interest in evaluating adipokines such as adiponectin and visfatin in several obesity-related diseases, including fatty liver disease and CVD, has been demonstrated [5,15]. Adiponectin is the most abundant peptide secreted by adipocytes. It was also found to be secreted from other cells, including skeletal and cardiac myocytes, in addition to endothelial cells. Reduction in adiponectin levels has a crucial role in obesity-related pathologies, such as insulin resistance, type 2 diabetes mellitus and CVD [16]. Although serum adiponectin levels were demonstrated to be similar in non-alcoholic fatty liver (NAFL) patients and controls based on liver histology, hypoadiponectinemia may exert an essential role in the progression from NAFL to non-alcoholic steatohepatitis (NASH) [17].

Visfatin is also secreted from adipocytes, as well as lymphocytes, neutrophils, monocytes, hepatocytes and pneumocytes [18]. Multiple pathways affected by visfatin include oxidative stress response, insulin resistance and inflammation [19–21]. A recently published meta-analysis evaluated serum visfatin levels in NAFLD, demonstrating no significant association [22]. Furthermore, increased visfatin levels were found to be associated with atherosclerotic disease and coronary artery disease (CAD), pathologies demonstrated to be among the main mortality causes in fatty liver disease [23–26].

Currently, the literature lacks studies evaluating serum adiponectin and visfatin levels in MAFLD patients using the newly defined criteria. Moreover, adiponectin and visfatin were both found to be associated with CVD, being responsible for most deaths among fatty liver disease patients, mainly due to ischemic heart disease [27,28]. Therefore, we conducted an observational cross-sectional study aiming to evaluate serum adiponectin and visfatin levels in MAFLD patients vs. controls, as well as their possible associations with cardiovascular parameters assessed by echocardiography and Doppler ultrasound. We hypothesized that adiponectin and visfatin can predict cardiovascular risk, mainly systolic and diastolic dysfunctions.

2. Materials and Methods

2.1. Study Participants and Setting

This is an observational cross-sectional study. Subjects were enrolled between January 2020 and September 2020 using non-probability consecutive sampling of eligible subjects. Inclusion criteria included subjects ≥ 18 and <65 years old. Patients admitted to the Clinical Emergency County Hospital of Cluj-Napoca, Romania, fulfilling the diagnostic criteria of MAFLD were included in the MAFLD group [9]. Hepatic steatosis was evaluated using both hepatic ultrasonography and SteatoTestTM (BioPredictive) simultaneously for the entire sample population (MAFLD patients and controls) at inclusion. Subjects had to present hepatic steatosis using both ultrasonography and SteatoTestTM (BioPredictive) in order to be included in the MAFLD group. Otherwise, they were excluded from the MAFLD group. Control participants were primarily healthy hospital staff not fulfilling the diagnostic criteria for MAFLD.

Exclusion criteria for both control and MAFLD groups included subjects with the presence of other secondary causes of hepatic steatosis evaluated by assessing alcohol consumption through AUDIT and CAGE questionnaires, use of hepatotoxic medications such as glucocorticoids, isoniazid, methotrexate, amiodarone and tamoxifen within 1 year from being enrolled in the study, positive hepatitis B or C virus serology, elevated ferritin concentration ≥ 1000 µg/L, significantly positive immunology titers for anti-smooth muscle antibody or antimitochondrial antibody, or a previous diagnosis of persistent secondary cause known for chronic liver disease. Moreover, individuals with benign or malignant liver tumor, coexistent liver disease, acute hemolytic diseases, acute inflammatory pathologies such as deep venous thrombosis, Ulcerative Colitis or Crohn's Disease, systemic lupus erythematosus, active malignancies, acute infections (dental, urinary, pulmonary, flu, COVID-19, etc.), active pulmonary exacerbations such as COPD exacerbation or asthma, failing to fast for a minimum of 12 h before blood sampling and refusing participation were excluded. The local ethical and research committee of "Iuliu Hatieganu" University of Medicine and Pharmacy Cluj-Napoca approved the performance of this study (no. 486/21 November 2019), which was conducted according to the 1975 Helsinki Declaration guidelines and revised in 2013. All included participants completed a written informed consent.

2.2. General Definitions

The diagnosis of MAFLD was based on the newly defined criteria [9]. The definition of hypertension was considered according to the 2020 International Society of Hypertension Global Hypertension Practice Guidelines [29]. The diagnosis of diabetes and prediabetes were determined according to the American Diabetes Association recommendations—Classification and Diagnosis of Diabetes: Standards of Medical Care in Diabetes (2021) [30]. Dyslipidemia was identified according to the National Cholesterol Education Program guidelines [31].

2.3. Hepatic Ultrasonography

Ultrasonographic evaluation of hepatic steatosis was performed using GE LOGIQ S7 Expert by an experienced physician who was blinded to the aims of the study, patients' diagnosis and labs. Subjects were requested to fast for a minimum of 8 h before performing the ultrasound evaluation, where a subcostal and intercostal approach was used to assess the liver parenchyma. Participants were evaluated in a supine position and in a modified, slightly oblique position with their right arm placed above their head and their right leg stretched. The following criteria were used in order to evaluate for hepatic steatosis: (1) ultrasonographic contrast between liver and right kidney parenchyma; (2) hepatic brightness; (3) ultrasound deep attenuation penetration into the deep portion of the liver and impaired diaphragmatic visualization; and (4) lumen narrowing and impaired intrahepatic vessels borders' visualization [32].

2.4. Echocardiography

A comprehensive echocardiographic assessment was conducted by a board-certified cardiologist who was blinded to the study aims, patients' diagnosis and labs, independent of the adipokines evaluation, using a GE Vivid q Ultrasound Machine, 11.2.0 b.40 software. The current recommendations and guidelines were used for measuring and interpreting our assessed parameters, including M-mode, 2-dimensional, conventional color and Doppler ultrasonography [33–38]. We used a dedicated software for automated calculation of end-systolic volume (ESV) and end-diastolic volume (EDV) from the 2- and 4-chamber apical views, as well as left ventricular ejection fraction (LVEF), while verification and correction of precision for the detected borders were conducted. Using apical 4-chamber views, we obtained Doppler-derived transmitral inflow profiles with a sample volume of 2 mm placed between the mitral leaflet tips. The early (E) and late (A) peak velocity phases of the mitral inflow were measured from the mitral inflow Doppler evaluation, while an automatic calculation was used for the E/A ratio. Moreover, also using the 4-chamber view, we calculated the LV myocardial velocities through Tissue Doppler imaging (TDI) with a sample volume being placed at the septal mitral annulus. We also calculated the early diastolic (e′) and late diastolic peak velocity phases using the pulsed-wave TDI, while the E/e′ ratio was automatically calculated.

2.5. Laboratory Analysis

We obtained blood samples through venipuncture and collected them in vacutainer tubes following 12 h of overnight fasting. We followed the recommended protocols for blood sampling and for analyzing blood samples.

2.5.1. Adipokines

For the adipokines' analysis (adiponectin and visfatin), peripheral blood was collected on a clot activator. Blood was transported to the Research Center for Functional Genomic, Biomedicine and Translational Medicine, "Iuliu Hatieganu" University of Medicine and Pharmacy, Cluj-Napoca, Romania within 30 min from sampling for centrifugation for 15 min at $1000\times g$ at 2~8 °C. The supernatant was collected to carry out the assay. Centrifuged blood samples were stored at −80 °C. The serum adiponectin analysis was performed using the BioVendor Adiponectin Human ELISA (Competitive) RD195023100 kit, while the serum visfatin analysis was performed using the Elabscience Human VF (Visfatin) ELISA Kit E-EL-H1763. All analyses were conducted as per the manufacturer's instructions.

2.5.2. FibroMax

Sera were separated and stored at 2 °C–8 °C for 1 day at most. Afterward, they were assayed for the ten serum biomarkers included in the FibroMax score. Adjustments for age, gender, weight and height of the achieved results were performed for obtaining the final score.

The serum levels of α2-macroglobulin, haptoglobin, apolipoprotein A1 were evaluated using nephelometry (BN ProSpec System from Siemens), while total bilirubin, gamma-glutamyltransferase (GGT), aspartate aminotransferase (AST), alanine aminotransferase (ALT), total cholesterol and triglycerides were assessed using spectrophotometry (Atellica from Siemens). Moreover, NaF/K2 oxalate spectrophotometry was used to assess plasma fasting glucose levels. Obtained values of the evaluated blood variables were completed into the BioPredictive network, where computed algorithms were performed.

2.6. Statistical Analysis

We used the R software environment for statistical computing and the graphics version 4.0.2 (R Foundation for Statistical Computing, Vienna, Austria) for carrying out the statistical analyses. Frequencies and percentages were used to report categorical data. For continuous data, normally distributed data were reported as mean (standard deviation, SD), while non-normally distributed data were reported as median (interquartile range, IQR). We used quantile–quantile plots to assess the normality of the distribution of the data. We used the *t*-test for independent samples of normally distributed data for comparing the clinical characteristics of the study population as per the categorized groups. Furthermore, the Wilcoxon rank-sum test was used for non-normally distributed data, while the chi-square test and Fisher's exact test were used for categorical data. We used Fisher's exact test in case expected frequencies were low, otherwise, we used chi-square tests. In order to evaluate the relationship between adiponectin and visfatin with several cardiovascular parameters, we performed Spearman's correlations, followed by univariate and multivariate linear regression models to control for confounding factors including MAFLD vs. controls, gender, diabetes, mean systolic blood pressure (SBP) (mmHg), mean diastolic blood pressure (DBP) (mmHg), low-density lipoprotein (LDL) and triglycerides. For all conducted linear models, we checked the assumptions of residual normality using a quantile–quantile plot, heteroskedasticity using standardized residual vs. fitted values, the presence of high leverage, high residuals, or high influential points using standardized residuals vs. hat-values vs. Cook's distance plot and the linearity relation of continuous variables with the outcome using component + residual plot. Moreover, we evaluated the presence of multicollinearity in multivariate models using correlation coefficients and variance inflation factors. We reported the regression results as model coefficients, 95% confidence interval (CI—computed with robust variance sandwich estimators in case of heteroskedasticity) and *p*-value. Furthermore, we performed multiple quantile regressions to better keep into account possible deviations from multiple linear model assumptions. Two-sided statistical tests were performed for all analyses. A *p*-value < 0.05 was considered to be statistically significant.

3. Results

3.1. General Characteristics and Laboratory Results

The subjects screened for eligibility were 252, out of which 172 were excluded with reasons as demonstrated in Figure 1. A total of 80 Caucasian participants were included in our study's final analysis. The participants' general characteristics are outlined in Table 1.

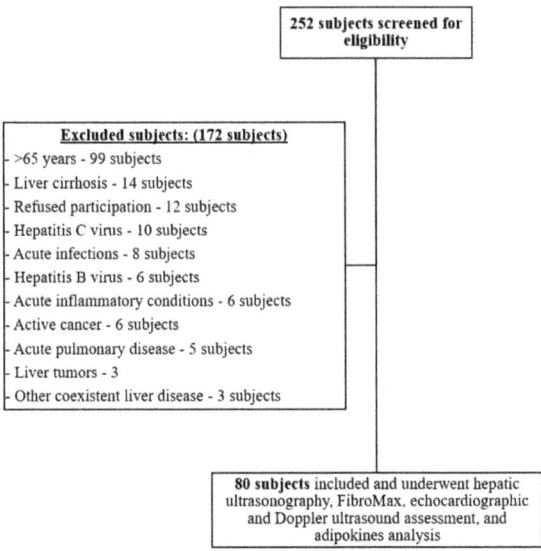

Figure 1. Flow diagram outlining the enrollment process of included and excluded participants.

Table 1. General characteristics of included participants.

Characteristic	Total (n = 80)	Control (n = 40)	MAFLD (n = 40)	p-Value
Age (years), median (IQR)	46 (30–57)	30 (27–42)	53.5 (48.75–59)	<0.001
Gender (male), n (%)	36/80 (45)	22 (55)	22 (55)	1
BMI, median (IQR)	26.4 (22.32–31.24)	22.29 (20.17–24.89)	30.78 (28.1–34.7)	<0.001
Waist circumference (cm), median (IQR)	96.5 (81.75–105.25)	82.5 (72–91.5)	104.5 (100–111)	<0.001
Metabolic syndrome, n (%)	33/80 (41.25)	2 (5)	31 (77.5)	<0.001
Diabetic, n (%)	16/80 (20)	0 (0)	16 (40)	<0.001
Impaired fasting glucose, n (%)	5/80 (6.25)	2 (5)	3 (7.5)	1
Hypertensive, n (%)	39/80 (48.75)	7 (17.5)	32 (80)	<0.001
SBP-mean (mmHg), median (IQR)	124.5 (116.38–137.25)	120.75 (112.5–126)	132.75 (122.38–147.88)	<0.001
DBP-mean (mmHg), median (IQR)	79 (74–84)	75.75 (71.25–79.12)	83 (78.38–89)	<0.001
MAP-mean (mmHg), median (IQR)	93.92 (89–101.88)	90.67 (84.42–94)	98.92 (92.79–108.62)	<0.001
Pulse pressure-mean (mmHg), median (IQR)	45.5 (41.38–52)	44.75 (40–49)	49.25 (42.38–58.5)	0.023
Pulse-mean (bpm), median (IQR)	77.5 (70.88–84.5)	79.5 (73.38–83.75)	76.75 (68–84.5)	0.366
Smoking history, n (%)				
Smoker:	16/80 (20)	8 (20)	8 (20)	0.963
Never smoked:	45/80 (56.25)	22 (55)	23 (57.5)	
Ex-smoker:	19/80 (23.75)	10 (25)	9 (22.5)	
LDL (mg/dL), median (IQR)	118 (90.5–158.5)	112.5 (84–140.75)	127 (99.75–166)	0.083
HDL (mg/dL), median (IQR)	48 (42.75–59.25)	54.5 (46.75–63)	44 (37.75–49.75)	<0.001
Triglycerides (mg/dL), median (IQR)	112 (79.5–154)	82.5 (69–103.5)	147.5 (115–184.5)	<0.001
Total cholesterol (mg/dL), median (IQR)	187.5 (151.75–219.25)	184 (152–215.25)	196 (146–230.25)	0.441
Fasting blood sugar (FBS) (mg/dL), median (IQR)	91 (86–100.25)	87 (82.75–91.25)	98 (89.5–123.75)	<0.001
Adiponectin (μg/mL), mean (SD)	10.92 (1.92)	11.28 (1.57)	10.56 (2.18)	0.097
Visfatin (ng/L), median (IQR)	16.91 (11.46–23.25)	14.94 (10.6–22.27)	18.18 (12.74–23.72)	0.26

IQR, interquartile range; MAFLD, metabolic-associated fatty liver disease; BMI, body mass index; DBP, diastolic blood pressure; HDL, high-density lipoprotein; LDL, low-density lipoprotein; MAP, mean arterial pressure; SBP, systolic blood pressure.

Participants were divided into 2 groups, MAFLD patients and controls, equally, with 40 subjects in each group with a total mean age of 46 (ranging from 30 to 57). Gender distribution was 44 females (55%) and 36 males (45%), with no statistically significant difference (p-value = 1). MAFLD patients had a higher BMI, larger waist circumference, presence of diabetes and hypertension compared to controls (p-value < 0.001). No significant difference was found regarding smoking history among both groups (p-value = 0.963). Blood pressure measurements, including SBP, DBP, mean arterial pressure and pulse pressure, were all significantly higher in MAFLD patients compared to controls, with a p-value of <0.001, <0.001, <0.001 and 0.023, respectively. High-density lipoprotein (HDL) levels were significantly lower in MAFLD patients with a p-value of <0.001, with no significant difference regarding LDL (p-value = 0.083) or total cholesterol (p-value = 0.441) levels.

3.2. Hepatic Steatosis and Fibrosis Evaluation

A summary of the obtained hepatic steatosis, liver fibrosis and FibroMax scores is outlined in Table S1. Although all MAFLD patients presented with hepatic steatosis on ultrasonography and SteatoTest, only one participant from the control group had hepatic steatosis but did not fulfill the rest of the criteria for MAFLD diagnosis. A significant difference was found in all evaluated hepatic steatosis (FLI and HSI), liver fibrosis (APRI, FIB-4, BARD and NAFLD fibrosis score) and FibroMax scores between MAFLD patients and controls.

3.3. Adipokine Levels

No significant difference was found between the levels of the two evaluated adipokines in MAFLD patients and controls, adiponectin and visfatin, with a p-value of 0.097 and 0.26, respectively.

3.4. Cardiovascular Assessment

Multiple echocardiographic and Doppler ultrasound parameters were evaluated as summarized in Table 2. Structural parameters included higher mean carotid intima medica thickness (CIMT) (p-value < 0.001), left atrial diameter (p-value < 0.001), left ventricular diameter (p-value = 0.002), right ventricular diameter (p-value = 0.003), left ventricular posterior wall thickness (LVPWT) (p-value < 0.001), interventricular septal wall thickness (p-value < 0.001) and interatrial septal wall thickness (p-value = 0.018) in MAFLD patients vs. controls. Functional parameters included higher left ventricular end systolic volume (LVESV) (p-value < 0.001), left ventricular end diastolic volume (LVEDV) (p-value < 0.001), stroke volume (p-value 0.027), cardiac output (p-value = 0.029), late diastolic peak velocity (A) (p-value < 0.001), E/A ratio (p-value < 0.001) and E/e' ratio (p-value = 0.004), as well as lower LVEF (p-value = 0.011), early diastolic peak velocity (E) (p-value < 0.001), early diastolic velocity (e') (p-value < 0.001), e'/a' (p-value < 0.001) in MAFLD patients vs. controls. No significant difference was observed in a' vales (p-value = 0.265).

Table 2. Echocardiographic and Doppler ultrasound cardiovascular parameters.

Characteristic	Total (n = 80)	Control (n = 40)	MAFLD (n = 40)	p-Value
CIMT-right (mm), median (IQR)	9 (7–10)	7 (6–9)	9.5 (8–11)	<0.001
CIMT-left (mm), median (IQR)	8.5 (7–10)	7 (6–8.25)	10 (8.75–11)	<0.001
CIMT-mean (mm), median (IQR)	8.5 (7–10)	7.25 (6.5–8.62)	9.75 (8.5–11)	<0.001
Left atrial diameter (mm), median (IQR)	31 (27–34)	29 (26–31)	34 (31–36.25)	<0.001
Left ventricular diameter (mm), median (IQR)	44 (39.75–48)	42 (38.75–44.25)	45 (43–49)	0.002
Right ventricular diameter (mm), median (IQR)	23 (21–25.25)	22 (20.75–24)	25 (22–27)	0.003
LVPWT (mm), median (IQR)	10 (8–10)	8 (8–9)	10 (10–11)	<0.001
Interventricular septal wall thickness (mm), median (IQR)	9 (8–10)	8.5 (8–9)	10 (9.75–11.25)	<0.001
Interatrial septal wall thickness (mm), median (IQR)	6 (5–7)	5 (5–7)	6 (6–7)	0.018
LVEDV (mL), median (IQR)	95 (78.5–114.25)	84 (73.75–104)	103 (92–121.75)	<0.001
LVESV (mL), median (IQR)	45 (36.75–56.75)	39 (32–47)	53.5 (43.75–62.75)	<0.001
Ejection fraction (EF) (%), median (IQR)	50 (46–56.25)	52.5 (48–57.5)	48.5 (45.75–52.5)	0.011
Stroke volume (mL), median (IQR)	51 (39–57)	44 (36.75–55.95)	53 (46.75–57.25)	0.027
Cardiac output, median (IQR)	3.52 (2.88–4.32)	3.22 (2.69–4.01)	3.79 (3.05–5.13)	0.029
Early diastolic peak velocity (E (m/s)), median (IQR)	0.74 (0.62–0.86)	0.8 (0.71–0.95)	0.66 (0.58–0.78)	<0.001
Late diastolic peak velocity (A (m/s)), median (IQR)	0.51 (0.43–0.73)	0.48 (0.42–0.57)	0.71 (0.5–0.79)	<0.001
Early diastolic velocity (e' (m/s)), median (IQR)	0.13 (0.11–0.17)	0.17 (0.14–0.2)	0.11 (0.09–0.13)	<0.001
Late diastolic velocity (a' (m/s)), median (IQR)	0.1 (0.07–0.14)	0.1 (0.07–0.13)	0.1 (0.08–0.16)	0.265
E/A ratio, median (IQR)	1.4 (0.98–1.8)	1.72 (1.32–1.98)	1.05 (0.76–1.42)	<0.001
e'/a' ratio, median (IQR)	1.46 (0.81–2.13)	1.67 (1.41–2.36)	0.93 (0.7–1.58)	<0.001
E/e' ratio, median (IQR)	5.38 (4.43–6.67)	5.05 (4.04–5.62)	5.96 (4.98–7.37)	0.004

IQR, interquartile range; MAFLD, metabolic-associated fatty liver disease; CIMT, carotid intima media thickness; LVEDV, left ventricular end diastolic volume; LVEF, left ventricular ejection fraction; LVESV, left ventricular end systolic volume; LVPWT, left ventricular posterior wall thickness; SBP, systolic blood pressure.

3.5. Adipokines and Cardiovascular Assessment

As demonstrated in Table S2, in the control group, visfatin levels were found to be inversely proportional and significantly associated with mean CIMT (p-value = 0.047), LVPWT (p-value = 0.003) and interventricular septal wall thickness (p-value = 0.008). Furthermore, in MAFLD patients, adiponectin was directly proportional and significantly related to A (p-value = 0.032), while, in controls, it was inversely proportional with LVEF (p-value = 0.039) and directly proportional with E (p-value = 0.003) and E/A ratio (p-value = 0.002). In all subjects, adiponectin levels were found to be significantly associated and inversely proportional with right ventricular diameter (p-value = 0.029) and LVPWT (p-value = 0.033) and directly proportional with E (p-value = 0.002).

We proceeded by assessing whether adiponectin and visfatin can be considered as potential biomarkers in evaluating E/A ratio, LVPWT, LVEF, CIMT and interventricular septal wall thickness by conducting several univariate and multivariate linear regression models adjusted for MAFLD, gender, diabetes, mean SBP (mmHg), mean DBP (mmHg), LDL and triglycerides, as reported in Table 3. No significant findings were demonstrated between adiponectin and LVPWT, nor between visfatin and LVPWT, CIMT and interventricular septal wall thickness in univariate and multivariate regression models. The association between adiponectin and E/A ratio was initially significant in the univariate linear regression analysis at 95% CI (0.0049–0.1331, p-value = 0.035). However, the significance was attenuated to non-significant levels after performing multivariate linear regression models. Interestingly, although the association between adiponectin and LVEF was not significant in the univariate analysis, significant values were reported after performing multivariate linear regression models with B-adjusted sandwich estimator of 95% CI ((-1.83)–(-0.22), p-value = 0.015) and with B-adjusted quantile regression estimator of 95% CI ((-1.97)–(-0.60), p-value = 0.011).

Table 3. Univariate and multivariate linear regression models and multivariate quantile regression models predicting E/A ratio, LVPWT, LVEF, CIMT (mean) and interventricular septal wall thickness in relation to adiponectin or visfatin, adjusted for MAFLD, sex, diabetes, SBP, DBP, LDL and triglycerides.

Dependent Variable	Predictor	B Unadjusted	(95% CI)	p-Value	R2	B Adjusted	(95% CI)	p-Value	B-Adjusted Sandwich	(95% CI)	p-Value	B-Adjusted Quantile	(95% CI)	p-Value
E/A ratio	Adiponectin (μg/mL)	0.069	(0.0049–0.1331)	0.035	0.056	0.0455	(−0.0148–0.1059)	0.137	0.0455	(−0.0191–0.1102)	0.172	0.04	(−0.4–0.7)	0.189
LVPWT	Adiponectin (μg/mL)	−0.15	(−0.31–0.01)	0.06	0.045	−0.02	(−0.15–0.11)	0.751	−0.02	(−0.16–0.12)	0.765	−0.03	(−0.19–0.09)	0.62
	Visfatin (ng/L)	0.0002	(−0.017–0.0173)	0.984	0	0	(−0.0125–0.0125)	0.995	0	(−0.0136–0.0136)	0.999	−0.0085	(−0.0293–0.0101)	0.263
LVEF	Adiponectin (μg/mL)	−0.52	(−1.31–0.28)	0.203	0.021	−1.03	(−1.92–−0.13)	0.026	−1.03	(−1.83–−0.22)	0.015	−1.39	(−1.97–−0.60)	0.011
CIMT (mean)	Visfatin (ng/L)	−0.0031	(−0.0283–0.0221)	0.809	0.001	−0.002	(−0.0234–0.0194)	0.852	−0.002	(−0.0203–0.0163)	0.831	−0.0028	(−0.0364–0.0141)	0.870
Interventricular septal wall thickness	Visfatin (ng/L)	−0.0012	(−0.0228–0.0204)	0.909	0	−0.0024	(−0.0186–0.0138)	0.766	−0.0024	(−0.0163–0.0115)	0.732	0.0013	(−0.0216–0.0096)	0.875

CIMT, carotid intima-media thickness; DBP, diastolic blood pressure; LDL, low-density lipoprotein; LVEF, left ventricular ejection fraction; LVPWT, left ventricular posterior wall thickness; MAFLD, metabolic associated fatty liver disease; SBP, systolic blood pressure.

4. Discussion

Several articles, including systematic reviews and meta-analyses evaluated adiponectin and visfatin levels in NAFLD [17,22]. However, so far, to the best of our knowledge, no studies have evaluated these adipokines in patients with MAFLD using the newly defined diagnosis criteria. Moreover, although decreased adiponectin levels and increased visfatin levels are known to be associated with several cardiovascular diseases, these parameters were not assessed in MAFLD patients for their possible use as potential biomarkers. Therefore, in this observational study, we aim to assess adiponectin and visfatin levels in MAFLD and their association with several cardiovascular parameters. We reported no significant difference in serum adiponectin and visfatin levels between MAFLD patients and controls. Moreover, a significant directly proportional association was reported between adiponectin and E/A ratio in the univariate linear regression analysis, while the association lost significance after adjustment using multivariate regression models. Although LVEF was not significantly associated with adiponectin in univariate analysis, interestingly, a significant inversely proportional association was demonstrated after adjustment using multivariate regression models.

Several results need to be further elaborated. In our study, we evaluated hepatic steatosis using hepatic ultrasonography, known to detect hepatocytes fat deposition only when >15–20% with a sensitivity ranging between 60 and 94% and specificity between 88 and 95% [39,40], along with SteatotestTM (Biopredictive), reported to provide a non-invasive and simple quantitative estimation of liver fat deposition, with an AUROC of 0.81 (95% CI 0.79–0.83, $p < 0.0001$) [41,42]. Currently, liver biopsy remains the gold standard for identifying hepatic steatosis and quantifying liver fibrosis. Nevertheless, it is an invasive procedure with possible complications.

Similar to currently published data, serum adiponectin and visfatin levels were not significantly different between MAFLD patients and controls in our study population. A systematic review and meta-analysis assessing adiponectin levels in NAFLD concluded that, according to liver histology, serum adiponectin levels were found to be similar in NAFL patients and controls [17]. However, the authors suggested that hypoadiponectinemia may exert a significant pathophysiological role in the progression from NAFL to NASH. Another systematic review and meta-analysis evaluated serum visfatin levels in NAFLD, concluding that visfatin levels were not found to be associated with NAFLD, whether biopsy-proven or ultrasound-diagnosed, presence or severity of hepatic steatosis, liver fibrosis, lobar inflammation, or NASH [22].

Although several published studies evaluated cardiovascular parameters in NAFLD patients, these data are scarce in the current literature involving MAFLD patients [43,44]. As reported in the current literature and the newly defined MAFLD criteria, patients with MAFLD present with metabolic dysregulations and cardiovascular risk factors, including metabolic syndrome, diabetes, hypertension and dyslipidemia [9,45]. These findings were also confirmed in our results. An interesting recently published study reported differences in cardiovascular mortality and all-cause mortality in patients with NAFLD and MAFLD, where MAFLD patients presented higher cardiovascular mortality and all-cause mortality risk [13]. Nevertheless, NAFLD per se was not associated with an increased risk of all-cause deaths after metabolic risk factors adjustment. Therefore, we believe that future studies should reevaluate important markers in MAFLD patients due to possible different results between both terms, perhaps elucidating pathogenic links related to the complex cardiovascular complications associated with MAFLD.

Age, sex and BMI are important factors that should be taken into account when interpreting echocardiographic findings. Several age-related changes have been demonstrated, including alterations in the left ventricular diastolic filling without significant age-related changes in resting left ventricular systolic function, mild increase in left ventricular mass and wall thickness, a slight decrease in left ventricular internal diastolic and systolic dimensions, especially in females, significant dilation in the left atrium in both sexes, thickening in valve leaflets and atrial septum [46]. Currently, optimal adjustment of echocardiographic parameters according to body size, especially in obese patients, remains challenging [47]. As we reported in our results in MAFLD patients, several alterations in echocardiographic parameters have been found in obese patients, including LA enlargement, left ventricular hypertrophy, as well as increased cardiac output and stroke volumes representing a physiological adaptation to increased metabolic needs [47].

In our study, we found a significant association between adiponectin and E/A ratio in univariate linear regression analysis, which lost significance after multivariate analysis. Similar to our findings, Norvik et al. conducted a cross-sectional study on 1165 women and 896 men without diabetes, reporting no significant association between adiponectin and E/A ratio [48]. On the other hand, Puchałowicz et al. reported that E/A was significantly positively associated with adiponectin in coronary artery disease patients [49]. Decreased adiponectin levels in obese subjects are linked with inflammation and increased cardiovascular risk [50–53].

Moreover, although LVEF was not significantly associated with adiponectin in the univariate analysis, interestingly, we found a significant inversely proportional association after conducting the multivariate regression analysis. Similarly, several published studies reported a significant inverse correlation between adiponectin and LVEF, where adiponectin levels increase significantly as LVEF worsens [54,55]. Although adiponectin levels are not predictive of the development of heart failure in humans, several human studies demonstrated that increased circulating adiponectin levels were linked to increased mortality in patients with chronic heart failure with reduced ejection fraction (HFrEF) [56–60].

Visfatin was proposed to be used as a biomarker for detecting atherosclerosis, endothelial dysfunction and vascular damage [25,26]. It is also considered to present potential prognostic value. Visfatin is a crucial player in promoting atherosclerosis and vascular inflammation. Elevated serum visfatin levels were observed in acute myocardial infarction patients and were linked to the earlier onset and higher incidence of major adverse cardiovascular events (MACE) [61]. Moreover, serum visfatin levels were positively related to CAD severity in patients with high SYNTAX scores [23]. As reported in a recently published systematic review, NAFLD patients were found to have an increased acute coronary syndrome (ACS) risk, mainly in Asian subjects, with inconsistent results in North American and European populations [62].

Our study has some limitations that need to be further discussed. Causality cannot be confirmed or negated between the reported associations due to the observational study design. We were not able to perform subgroup analyses due to the enrolled modest sample size; further, adjustments using multivariate analysis might not account for some differences in basic characteristics. The increased values of hepatic steatosis and liver fibrosis scores, as well as changes in the evaluated echocardiographic parameters can partially be attributed to the increased age of MAFLD patients compared to controls. This can be due to differences in recruitment strategies, because our controls were mainly hospital staff not known to have medical illnesses. However, we partially corrected for these differences by including the MAFLD variable in our multivariate linear regression models, which is partially correlated (multicollinear) with BMI and age. Nevertheless, these adjustments cannot completely control for said differences. Furthermore, the study being observational, residual confounding can still persist. In addition, since the systolic and diastolic functions are measured by different parameters, analyzing them can increase the family-wise error rate. We cannot generalize our results as this is a single-center study conducted only on Caucasian subjects. Another limit in generalization is due to the exclusion of patients >65 years old, in order to limit confounding of comorbidities, being known that MAFLD population is relatively older. Histopathological assessment of hepatic steatosis by liver biopsy, the current gold standard, was not performed. Therefore, results should be interpreted with caution due to the above-mentioned limitations.

Our study also has several important strengths. Hepatic steatosis was assessed by combining hepatic ultrasonography and SteatoTestTM (Biopredictive), therefore improving the accuracy of predicting hepatic steatosis. Furthermore, the new criteria for MAFLD, reported to be able to identify fatty liver disease patients with increased disease progression risk, were used in our study [45]. To the best of our knowledge, this is the first study to assess serum adiponectin and visfatin levels in MAFLD patients, as well as the first to include comprehensive cardiovascular echocardiographic and Doppler ultrasound parameters and their association with adiponectin and visfatin. Due to the increasing worldwide prevalence of metabolic disorders, including fatty liver disease, as well as the associated increased CV risk, being associated with increased morbidity and mortality, we believe that the findings of our study are of clinical significance.

5. Conclusions

No significant association between serum adiponectin and visfatin levels was observed in MAFLD patients vs. controls. Despite the E/A ratio being significantly associated with adiponectin in the univariate analysis, this association was attenuated after performing multivariate linear regression models. Interestingly, although adiponectin levels were not associated with LVEF in the univariate analysis, a significant inversely proportional association was observed after the multivariate linear regression analysis. However, adiponectin and visfatin levels did not predict left ventricular posterior wall thickness, while visfatin levels did not predict CIMT and interventricular septal wall thickness.

In order to confirm our demonstrated results, it is necessary to conduct further observational studies involving a larger sample size on populations from different backgrounds. Hence, adiponectin can possibly play an important role in identifying incipient cardiovascular disease in MAFLD patients through the reduction and prevention of associated cardiovascular morbidity and mortality.

Supplementary Materials: The following are available online at https://www.mdpi.com/article/10.3390/jcm10215194/s1, Table S1: Hepatic steatosis and fibrosis evaluation of included participants. Table S2: Spearman's correlation coefficient analyses assessing the relation between adiponectin and visfatin levels with echocardiographic and Doppler ultrasound cardiovascular parameters.

Author Contributions: Conceptualization, A.I. and D.L.D.; methodology, A.I., D.-C.L., S.-L.P. and D.L.D.; software, A.I. and D.-C.L.; formal analysis, A.I. and D.-C.L.; investigation, A.I., M.S., L.B., S.-L.P. and B.A.C.; resources, A.I. and D.L.D.; data curation, A.I.; writing—original draft preparation, A.I.; writing—review and editing, M.S., L.B., D.-C.L., S.-L.P. and B.A.C.; visualization, A.I.; supervision, I.B.-N., D.M.O. and D.L.D.; project administration, A.I.; funding acquisition, A.I. All authors have read and agreed to the published version of the manuscript.

Funding: This study was partially funded by the doctoral research project grant received by A.I. from "Iuliu Hatieganu" University of Medicine and Pharmacy Cluj-Napoca, contract no. 1529/35/18.01.2019.

Institutional Review Board Statement: The study was conducted according to the guidelines of the Declaration of Helsinki and approved by the Ethics Committee of "Iuliu Hatieganu" University of Medicine and Pharmacy Cluj-Napoca (no. 486/21 November 2019).

Informed Consent Statement: Informed consent was obtained from all subjects involved in the study.

Data Availability Statement: Data supporting the reported results can be obtained by contacting A.I. or S.L.P.

Acknowledgments: Performed FibroMax analyses were supported by BioPredictive.

Conflicts of Interest: The authors declare no conflict of interest.

References

1. Dumitrascu, D.L.; Neuman, M.G. Non-alcoholic fatty liver disease: An update on diagnosis. *Clujul Med.* **2018**, *91*, 147–150. [CrossRef]
2. Sporea, I.; Popescu, A.; Dumitrașcu, D.; Brisc, C.; Nedelcu, L.; Trifan, A.; Gheorghe, L.; Braticevici, C.F. Nonalcoholic Fatty Liver Disease: Status Quo. *J. Gastrointest. Liver Dis.* **2018**, *27*, 439–448. [CrossRef]
3. Mantovani, A.; Scorletti, E.; Mosca, A.; Alisi, A.; Byrne, C.D.; Targher, G. Complications, morbidity and mortality of nonalcoholic fatty liver disease. *Metabolism* **2020**, *111*, 154170. [CrossRef] [PubMed]

4. Francque, S.M.; van der Graaff, D.; Kwanten, W. Non-alcoholic fatty liver disease and cardiovascular risk: Pathophysiological mechanisms and implications. *J. Hepatol.* **2016**, *65*, 425–443. [CrossRef] [PubMed]
5. Mirza, M.S. Obesity, Visceral Fat, and NAFLD: Querying the Role of Adipokines in the Progression of Nonalcoholic Fatty Liver Disease. *ISRN Gastroenterol.* **2011**, *2011*, 592404. [CrossRef] [PubMed]
6. Ando, Y.; Jou, J.H. Nonalcoholic Fatty Liver Disease and Recent Guideline Updates. *Clin. Liver Dis.* **2021**, *17*, 23–28. [CrossRef]
7. European Association for the Study of the Liver (EASL); European Association for the Study of Diabetes (EASD); European Association for the Study of Obesity (EASO). EASL–EASD–EASO Clinical Practice Guidelines for the management of non-alcoholic fatty liver disease. *J. Hepatol.* **2016**, *64*, 1388–1402. [CrossRef]
8. Eslam, M.; Newsome, P.N.; Sarin, S.K.; Anstee, Q.M.; Targher, G.; Romero-Gomez, M.; Zelber-Sagi, S.; Wong, V.W.-S.; Dufour, J.-F.; Schattenberg, J.M.; et al. A new definition for metabolic dysfunction-associated fatty liver disease: An international expert consensus statement. *J. Hepatol.* **2020**, *73*, 202–209. [CrossRef]
9. Eslam, M.; Sanyal, A.J.; George, J.; Neuschwander-Tetri, B.; Tiribelli, C.; Kleiner, D.E.; Brunt, E.; Bugianesi, E.; Yki-Järvinen, H.; Grønbæk, H.; et al. MAFLD: A Consensus-Driven Proposed Nomenclature for Metabolic Associated Fatty Liver Disease. *Gastroenterology* **2020**, *158*, 1999–2014. [CrossRef]
10. Wong, C.; Lim, J.K. The Association Between Nonalcoholic Fatty Liver Disease and Cardiovascular Disease Outcomes. *Clin. Liver Dis.* **2018**, *12*, 39–44. [CrossRef]
11. Targher, G.; Marra, F.; Marchesini, G. Increased risk of cardiovascular disease in non-alcoholic fatty liver disease: Causal effect or epiphenomenon? *Diabetologia* **2008**, *51*, 1947–1953. [CrossRef]
12. Ismaiel, A.; Dumitraşcu, D.L. Cardiovascular Risk in Fatty Liver Disease: The Liver-Heart Axis—Literature Review. *Front. Med.* **2019**, *6*, 202. [CrossRef]
13. Kim, D.; Konyn, P.; Sandhu, K.K.; Dennis, B.B.; Cheung, A.C.; Ahmed, A. Metabolic dysfunction-associated fatty liver disease is associated with increased all-cause mortality in the United States. *J. Hepatol.* **2021**. [CrossRef]
14. Lee, H.; Lee, Y.-H.; Kim, S.U.; Kim, H.C. Metabolic Dysfunction-Associated Fatty Liver Disease and Incident Cardiovascular Disease Risk: A Nationwide Cohort Study. *Clin. Gastroenterol. Hepatol.* **2021**, *19*, 2138–2147.e10. [CrossRef] [PubMed]
15. Funcke, J.-B.; Scherer, P.E. Beyond adiponectin and leptin: Adipose tissue-derived mediators of inter-organ communication. *J. Lipid Res.* **2019**, *60*, 1648–1697. [CrossRef] [PubMed]
16. Achari, A.E.; Jain, S.K. Adiponectin, a Therapeutic Target for Obesity, Diabetes, and Endothelial Dysfunction. *Int. J. Mol. Sci.* **2017**, *18*, 1321. [CrossRef] [PubMed]
17. Polyzos, S.A.; Toulis, K.A.; Goulis, D.G.; Zavos, C.; Kountouras, J. Serum total adiponectin in nonalcoholic fatty liver disease: A systematic review and meta-analysis. *Metabolism* **2011**, *60*, 313–326. [CrossRef]
18. Samal, B.; Sun, Y.; Stearns, G.; Xie, C.; Suggs, S.; Mcniece, I. Cloning and characterization of the cDNA encoding a novel human pre-B-cell colony-enhancing factor. *Mol. Cell. Biol.* **1994**, *14*, 1431–1437. [CrossRef]
19. Wang, T.; Zhang, X.; Bheda, P.; Revollo, J.R.; Imai, S.-I.; Wolberger, C. Structure of Nampt/PBEF/visfatin, a mammalian NAD+ biosynthetic enzyme. *Nat. Struct. Mol. Biol.* **2006**, *13*, 661–662. [CrossRef]
20. Revollo, J.R.; Grimm, A.A.; Imai, S.-I. The NAD Biosynthesis Pathway Mediated by Nicotinamide Phosphoribosyltransferase Regulates Sir2 Activity in Mammalian Cells. *J. Biol. Chem.* **2004**, *279*, 50754–50763. [CrossRef]
21. Adolph, T.E.; Grander, C.; Grabherr, F.; Tilg, H. Adipokines and Non-Alcoholic Fatty Liver Disease: Multiple Interactions. *Int. J. Mol. Sci.* **2017**, *18*, 1649. [CrossRef]
22. Ismaiel, A.; Leucuta, D.-C.; Popa, S.-L.; Dumitrascu, D. Serum Visfatin Levels in Nonalcoholic Fatty Liver Disease and Liver Fibrosis: Systematic Review and Meta-Analysis. *J. Clin. Med.* **2021**, *10*, 3029. [CrossRef] [PubMed]
23. Duman, H.; Özyıldız, A.G.; Bahçeci, I.; Duman, H.; Uslu, A.; Ergül, E. Serum visfatin level is associated with complexity of coronary artery disease in patients with stable angina pectoris. *Ther. Adv. Cardiovasc. Dis.* **2019**, *13*, 1753944719880448. [CrossRef] [PubMed]
24. Zheng, L.-Y.; Xu, X.; Wan, R.-H.; Xia, S.; Lu, J.; Huang, Q. Association between serum visfatin levels and atherosclerotic plaque in patients with type 2 diabetes. *Diabetol. Metab. Syndr.* **2019**, *11*, 1–7. [CrossRef] [PubMed]
25. Hognogi, L.D.M.; Simiti, L.V. The cardiovascular impact of visfatin—An inflammation predictor biomarker in metabolic syndrome. *Clujul Med.* **2016**, *89*, 322–326. [CrossRef]
26. Romacho, T.; Sánchez-Ferrer, C.F.; Peiro, C. Visfatin/Nampt: An Adipokine with Cardiovascular Impact. *Mediat. Inflamm.* **2013**, *2013*, 946427. [CrossRef] [PubMed]
27. Targher, G.; Day, C.P.; Bonora, E. Risk of Cardiovascular Disease in Patients with Nonalcoholic Fatty Liver Disease. *N. Engl. J. Med.* **2010**, *363*, 1341–1350. [CrossRef]
28. Byrne, C.D.; Targher, G. NAFLD: A multisystem disease. *J. Hepatol.* **2015**, *62* (Suppl. 1), S47–S64. [CrossRef]
29. Unger, T.; Borghi, C.; Charchar, F.; Khan, N.A.; Poulter, N.R.; Prabhakaran, D.; Ramirez, A.; Schlaich, M.; Stergiou, G.S.; Tomaszewski, M.; et al. 2020 International Society of Hypertension Global Hypertension Practice Guidelines. *Hypertension* **2020**, *75*, 1334–1357. [CrossRef]
30. American Diabetes Association. 2. Classification and Diagnosis of Diabetes: Standards of Medical Care in Diabetes—2021. *Diabetes Care* **2020**, *44* (Suppl. 1), S15–S33. [CrossRef]
31. Grundy, S.M. Third Report of the National Cholesterol Education Program (NCEP) Expert Panel on Detection, Evaluation, and Treatment of High Blood Cholesterol in Adults (Adult Treatment Panel III) final report. *Circulation* **2002**, *106*, 3143–3421.

32. Pan, J.-J.; Fisher-Hoch, S.P.; Chen, C.; Feldstein, A.E.; McCormick, J.B.; Rahbar, M.H.; Beretta, L.; Fallon, M.B. Burden of nonalcoholic fatty liver disease and advanced fibrosis in a Texas Hispanic community cohort. *World J. Hepatol.* **2015**, *7*, 1586–1594. [CrossRef]
33. Lang, R.M.; Bierig, M.; Devereux, R.B.; Flachskampf, F.A.; Foster, E.; Pellikka, P.A.; Picard, M.; Roman, M.J.; Seward, J.B.; Shanewise, J.S. Recommendations for chamber quantification. *Eur. J. Echocardiogr.* **2006**, *7*, 79–108. [CrossRef] [PubMed]
34. Lancellotti, P.; Tribouilloy, C.; Hagendorff, A.; Popescu, B.A.; Edvardsen, T.; Pierard, L.A.; Badano, L.; Zamorano, J.L. Recommendations for the echocardiographic assessment of native valvular regurgitation: An executive summary from the European Association of Cardiovascular Imaging. *Eur. Hear. J. Cardiovasc. Imaging* **2013**, *14*, 611–644. [CrossRef] [PubMed]
35. Nagueh, S.F.; Smiseth, O.A.; Appleton, C.P.; Byrd, B.F., 3rd; Dokainish, H.; Edvardsen, T.; Flachskampf, F.A.; Gillebert, T.; Klein, A.L.; Lancellotti, P.; et al. Recommendations for the Evaluation of Left Ventricular Diastolic Function by Echocardiography: An Update from the American Society of Echocardiography and the European Association of Cardiovascular Imaging. *J. Am. Soc. Echocardiogr.* **2016**, *29*, 277–314. [CrossRef]
36. Vijayaraghavan, G.; Sivasankaran, S. Global longitudinal strain: A practical step-by-step approach to longitudinal strain imaging. *J. Indian Acad. Echocardiogr. Cardiovasc. Imaging* **2020**, *4*, 22. [CrossRef]
37. Muraru, D.; Cucchini, U.; Mihăilă, S.; Miglioranza, M.H.; Aruta, P.; Cavalli, G.; Cecchetto, A.; Padayattil-Josè, S.; Peluso, D.; Iliceto, S.; et al. Left Ventricular Myocardial Strain by Three-Dimensional Speckle-Tracking Echocardiography in Healthy Subjects: Reference Values and Analysis of Their Physiologic and Technical Determinants. *J. Am. Soc. Echocardiogr.* **2014**, *27*, 858–871.e1. [CrossRef]
38. Reisner, S.A.; Lysyansky, P.; Agmon, Y.; Mutlak, D.; Lessick, J.; Friedman, Z. Global longitudinal strain: A novel index of left ventricular systolic function. *J. Am. Soc. Echocardiogr.* **2004**, *17*, 630–633. [CrossRef]
39. Lupsor-Platon, M.; Stefanescu, H.; Muresan, D.; Florea, M.; Szasz, M.E.; Maniu, A.; Badea, R. Noninvasive assessment of liver ste-atosis using ultrasound methods. *Med. Ultrason.* **2014**, *16*, 236–245.
40. Joy, D.; Thava, V.R.; Scott, B.B. Diagnosis of fatty liver disease: Is biopsy necessary? *Eur. J. Gastroenterol. Hepatol.* **2003**, *15*, 539–543. [CrossRef]
41. Poynard, T.; Ratziu, V.; Naveau, S.; Thabut, D.; Charlotte, F.; Messous, D.; Capron, D.; Abella, A.; Massard, J.; Ngo, Y.; et al. The diagnostic value of biomarkers (SteatoTest) for the prediction of liver steatosis. *Comp. Hepatol.* **2005**, *4*, 10. [CrossRef]
42. Lassailly, G.; Caiazzo, R.; Hollebecque, A.; Buob, D.; Leteurtre, E.; Arnalsteen, L.; Louvet, A.; Pigeyre, M.; Raverdy, V.; Verkindt, H.; et al. Validation of noninvasive biomarkers (FibroTest, SteatoTest, and NashTest) for prediction of liver injury in patients with morbid obesity. *Eur. J. Gastroenterol. Hepatol.* **2011**, *23*, 499–506. [CrossRef] [PubMed]
43. Bonci, E.; Chiesa, C.; Versacci, P.; Anania, C.; Silvestri, L.; Pacifico, L. Association of Nonalcoholic Fatty Liver Disease with Subclinical Cardiovascular Changes: A Systematic Review and Meta-Analysis. *BioMed Res. Int.* **2015**, *2015*, 213737. [CrossRef] [PubMed]
44. Wijarnpreecha, K.; Lou, S.; Panjawatanan, P.; Cheungpasitporn, W.; Pungpapong, S.; Lukens, F.J.; Ungprasert, P. Association between diastolic cardiac dysfunction and nonalcoholic fatty liver disease: A systematic review and meta-analysis. *Dig. Liver Dis.* **2018**, *50*, 1166–1175. [CrossRef] [PubMed]
45. Lin, S.; Huang, J.; Wang, M.; Kumar, R.; Liu, Y.; Liu, S.; Wu, Y.; Wang, X.; Zhu, Y. Comparison of MAFLD and NAFLD diagnostic criteria in real world. *Liver Int.* **2020**, *40*, 2082–2089. [CrossRef]
46. Kitzman, D.W. Normal Age-Related Changes in the Heart: Relevance to Echocardiography in the Elderly. *Am. J. Geriatr. Cardiol.* **2000**, *9*, 311–320. [CrossRef]
47. Singh, M.; Sethi, A.; Mishra, A.K.; Subrayappa, N.K.; Stapleton, D.D.; Pellikka, P.A. Echocardiographic Imaging Challenges in Obesity: Guideline Recommendations and Limitations of Adjusting to Body Size. *J. Am. Heart Assoc.* **2020**, *9*, e014609. [CrossRef]
48. Norvik, J.V.; Schirmer, H.; Ytrehus, K.; Jenssen, T.G.; Zykova, S.N.; Eggen, A.E.; Eriksen, B.O.; Solbu, M.D. Low adiponectin is associated with diastolic dysfunction in women: A cross-sectional study from the Tromsø Study. *BMC Cardiovasc. Disord.* **2017**, *17*, 1–10. [CrossRef] [PubMed]
49. Puchałowicz, K.; Kłoda, K.; Dziedziejko, V.; Rać, M.; Wojtarowicz, A.; Chlubek, D.; Safranow, K. Association of Adiponectin, Leptin and Resistin Plasma Concentrations with Echocardiographic Parameters in Patients with Coronary Artery Disease. *Diagnostics* **2021**, *11*, 1774. [CrossRef]
50. Francisco, C.; Neves, J.S.; Falcão-Pires, I.; Leite-Moreira, A. Can Adiponectin Help us to Target Diastolic Dysfunction? *Cardiovasc. Drugs Ther.* **2016**, *30*, 635–644. [CrossRef]
51. Engeli, S.; Feldpausch, M.; Gorzelniak, K.; Hartwig, F.; Heintze, U.; Janke, J.; Möhlig, M.; Pfeiffer, A.F.; Luft, F.C.; Sharma, A.M. Association Between Adiponectin and Mediators of Inflammation in Obese Women. *Diabetes* **2003**, *52*, 942–947. [CrossRef]
52. Akoumianakis, I.; Antoniades, C. The interplay between adipose tissue and the cardiovascular system: Is fat always bad? *Cardiovasc. Res.* **2017**, *113*, 999–1008. [CrossRef] [PubMed]
53. Oh, A.; Okazaki, R.; Sam, F.; Valero-Munoz, M. Heart Failure With Preserved Ejection Fraction and Adipose Tissue: A Story of Two Tales. *Front. Cardiovasc. Med.* **2019**, *6*, 110. [CrossRef] [PubMed]
54. Tengiz, I.; Turk, U.O.; Alioglu, E.; Kirilmaz, B.; Tamer, G.S.; Tuzun, N.; Ercan, E. The relationship between adiponectin, NT-pro-BNP and left ventricular ejection fraction in non-cachectic patients with systolic heart failure: An observational study. *Anadolu Kardiyol. Dergisi/Anatol. J. Cardiol.* **2013**, *13*, 221–226. [CrossRef]

55. Oztürk, M.; Dursunoğlu, D.; Göksoy, H.; Rota, S.; Gür, S. Evaluation of serum adiponectin levels in patients with heart failure and relationship with functional capacity. *Turk Kardiyol. Dern. Ars. Turk Kardiyol. Dern. Yayin Organidir* **2009**, *37*, 384–390.
56. Frankel, D.S.; Vasan, R.S.; D'Agostino, R.B.; Benjamin, E.; Levy, D.; Wang, T.; Meigs, J.B. Resistin, Adiponectin, and Risk of Heart Failure: The Framingham Offspring Study. *J. Am. Coll. Cardiol.* **2009**, *53*, 754–762. [CrossRef]
57. Kistorp, C.; Faber, J.; Galatius, S.; Gustafsson, F.; Frystyk, J.; Flyvbjerg, A.; Hildebrandt, P. Plasma Adiponectin, Body Mass Index, and Mortality in Patients With Chronic Heart Failure. *Circulation* **2005**, *112*, 1756–1762. [CrossRef]
58. George, J.; Patal, S.; Wexler, D.; Sharabi, Y.; Peleg, E.; Kamari, Y.; Grossman, E.; Sheps, D.; Keren, G.; Roth, A. Circulating adiponectin concentrations in patients with congestive heart failure. *Heart* **2006**, *92*, 1420–1424. [CrossRef]
59. Tamura, T.; Furukawa, Y.; Taniguchi, R.; Sato, Y.; Ono, K.; Horiuchi, H.; Nakagawa, Y.; Kita, T.; Kimura, T. Serum Adiponectin Level as an Independent Predictor of Mortality in Patients With Congestive Heart Failure. *Circ. J.* **2007**, *71*, 623–630. [CrossRef]
60. Tanaka, K.; Wilson, R.M.; Essick, E.E.; Duffen, J.L.; Scherer, P.E.; Ouchi, N.; Sam, F. Effects of Adiponectin on Calcium-Handling Proteins in Heart Failure With Preserved Ejection Fraction. *Circ. Heart Fail.* **2014**, *7*, 976–985. [CrossRef]
61. Zheng, M.; Lu, N.; Ren, M.; Chen, H. Visfatin associated with major adverse cardiovascular events in patients with acute myocardial infarction. *BMC Cardiovasc. Disord.* **2020**, *20*, 271. [CrossRef] [PubMed]
62. Ismaiel, A.; Popa, S.-L.; Dumitrascu, D.L. Acute Coronary Syndromes and Nonalcoholic Fatty Liver Disease: "Un Affaire de Coeur". *Can. J. Gastroenterol. Hepatol.* **2020**, *2020*, 8825615. [CrossRef] [PubMed]

MDPI
St. Alban-Anlage 66
4052 Basel
Switzerland
Tel. +41 61 683 77 34
Fax +41 61 302 89 18
www.mdpi.com

Journal of Clinical Medicine Editorial Office
E-mail: jcm@mdpi.com
www.mdpi.com/journal/jcm

www.ingramcontent.com/pod-product-compliance
Lightning Source LLC
LaVergne TN
LVHW070043120526
838202LV00101B/423